Primary Care Dermatology

Editor

GEORGE G.A. PUJALTE

PRIMARY CARE: CLINICS IN OFFICE PRACTICE

www.primarycare.theclinics.com

Consulting Editor
JOEL J. HEIDELBAUGH

December 2015 • Volume 42 • Number 4

ELSEVIER

1600 John F. Kennedy Boulevard • Suite 1800 • Philadelphia, Pennsylvania, 19103-2899

http://www.theclinics.com

PRIMARY CARE: CLINICS IN OFFICE PRACTICE Volume 42, Number 4
December 2015 ISSN 0095-4543, ISBN-13: 978-0-323-40266-8

Editor: Jessica McCool
Developmental Editor: Colleen Viola

Primary Care: Clinics in Office Practice (ISSN: 0095–4543) is published quarterly by Elsevier Inc., 360 Park Avenue South, New York, NY 10010-1710. Months of issue are March, June, September, and December. Periodicals postage paid at New York, NY and additional mailing offices. Subscription prices are $225.00 per year (US individuals), $392.00 (US institutions), $115.00 (US students), $275.00 (Canadian individuals), $444.00 (Canadian institutions), $175.00 (Canadian students), $345.00 (international individuals), $444.00 (international institutions), and $175.00 (international students). Foreign air speed delivery is included in all *Clinics* subscription prices. All prices are subject to change without notice. POSTMASTER: Send address changes to *Primary Care: Clinics in Office Practice*, Elsevier Periodicals Customer Service, 11830 Westline Industrial Drive, St. Louis, MO 63146. Customer Service Health Sciences Division, Subscription Customer Service, 3251 Riverport Lane, Maryland Heights, MO 63043. **Customer Service: 1-800-654-2452 (U.S. and Canada); 314-447-8871 (outside U.S. and Canada). Fax: 314-447-8029. E-mail: journalscustomerservice-usa@elsevier.com (for print support); journalsonlinesupport-usa@elsevier.com (for online support).**

Reprints. For copies of 100 or more, of articles in this publication, please contact the Commercial Reprints Department, Elsevier Inc., 360 Park Avenue South, New York, NY 10010-1710. Tel. 212-633-3874; Fax: 212-633-3820; E-mail: reprints@elsevier.com.

Primary Care: Clinics in Office Practice is covered in *MEDLINE/PubMed (Index Medicus)* and *EMBASE/ Excerpta Medica, Current Contents/Clinical Medicine, and ISI/BIOMED.*

Contributors

CONSULTING EDITOR

JOEL J. HEIDELBAUGH, MD, FAAFP, FACG
Clinical Professor, Departments of Family Medicine and Urology; Clerkship Director, Department of Family Medicine, University of Michigan Medical School, Ann Arbor, Michigan; Ypsilanti Health Center, Ypsilanti, Michigan

EDITOR

GEORGE G.A. PUJALTE, MD, FACSM
Assistant Professor, Family Medicine and Sports Medicine, Department of Family Medicine, Mayo Clinic, Jacksonville, Florida

AUTHORS

ISABELLA AHANOGBE, MD
Manning Regional Health Care Center, Manning, Iowa

PAUL A. BOTROS, MD
Department of Family and Community Medicine, Penn State Milton S. Hershey Medical Center, Hershey, Pennsylvania

JESSICA F. BUTTS, MD
Assistant Professor, Departments of Family and Community Medicine and Orthopedics and Rehabilitation, Penn State Milton S. Hershey Medical Center, Hershey, Pennsylvania

IRFAN DADABHOY, MD
PGY-2, Penn State Hershey Family Medicine Residency Program, Hershey, Pennsylvania

HAROLD F. FARBER, MD
Board Certified Dermatologist; Director, Center for Dermatology, Laser, and Cosmetic Surgery, Director, Psoriasis Infusion and Treatment Center, Philadelphia, Pennsylvania

ALDE CARLO P. GAVINO, MD
Assistant Professor of Dermatology, Dell Medical School, The University of Texas at Austin, Austin, Texas

FADI IBRAHIM, MD
Resident, Family Medicine, Mount Sinai Hospital, Chicago, Illinois

NWAMAKA ISAMAH, MD
PGY-3 Family Medicine Resident, Penn State Hershey Family and Community Medicine Residency Program, Department of Family Medicine, Penn State Milton S. Hershey Medical Center, Hershey, Pennsylvania

LENA JAFILAN, MD
Department of Family and Community Medicine, Resident Physician, Penn State Milton S. Hershey Medical Center, Hershey, Pennsylvania

CHARIS JAMES, MD, MPH
Department of Family and Community Medicine, Resident Physician, Penn State Milton S. Hershey Medical Center, Hershey, Pennsylvania

NEHA KAUSHIK, MD
PGY-3 Family Medicine Resident, Community Medicine Residency Program, Department of Family Medicine, Penn State Milton S. Hershey Medical Center, Hershey, Pennsylvania

TARIQ KHAN, MD
Resident, Family Medicine, Mount Sinai Hospital, Chicago, Illinois

KATHERINE JANE LANGLEY, MD
Resident Physician, Department of Emergency Medicine, West Virginia University, Morgantown, West Virginia

MIGUEL A. LINARES, MD
Primary Care Sports Medicine Fellow, Henry Ford Hospital, Detroit, Michigan

AARON J. MONSEAU, MD
Assistant Professor, Department of Emergency Medicine, West Virginia University, Morgantown, West Virginia

SAHIL MULLICK, MD
Department of Family Medicine, Creighton University Medical Center, Omaha, Nebraska

PARMINDER NIZRAN, MD, CCFP
Albion Family Clinic and Walkin, Etobicoke, Ontario, Canada

REBECCA M. NORTHWAY, MD
Clinical Instructor, Internal Medicine-Pediatrics, University of Michigan Medical Hospital, University of Michigan, Ann Arbor, Michigan

CAYCE ONKS, DO, MS, ATC
Assistant Professor, Departments of Family & Community Medicine and Orthopaedics and Rehabilitation, Penn State Milton S. Hershey Medical Center, Hershey, Pennsylvania

SHAWN PHILLIPS, MD, MSPT
Assistant Professor, Departments of Family and Community Medicine and Orthopedics and Rehabilitation, Penn State Milton S. Hershey Medical Center, Hershey, Pennsylvania

GEORGE G.A. PUJALTE, MD, FACSM
Assistant Professor, Family Medicine and Sports Medicine, Department of Family Medicine, Mayo Clinic, Jacksonville, Florida

PRIYA RAMDASS, MD
Department of Family and Community Medicine, Mount Sinai Medical Center, Chicago, Illinois

ZEBULA M. REED, MD
Resident Physician, Department of Emergency Medicine, West Virginia University, Morgantown, West Virginia

STEPHANIE T. REESE, DO
Division of Primary Care, Family Medicine, Mayo Clinic Health System, Waycross, Georgia

ELIZABETH SEIVERLING, MD
Assistant Professor, Department of Dermatology, Penn State Hershey Dermatology, Hershey, Pennsylvania

MATTHEW SILVIS, MD
Penn State Primary Care Sports Medicine Fellowship, Associate Professor, Departments of Family and Community Medicine and Orthopedics and Rehabilitation, Penn State Milton S. Hershey Medical Center, Hershey, Pennsylvania

GARY TSAI, MD
Department of Family and Community Medicine, Penn State Milton S. Hershey Medical Center, Hershey, Pennsylvania

JAMES RORY J. TUCKER, MD
Assistant Professor of Family and Community Medicine, and Orthopedics and Rehabilitation, Department of Family and Community Medicine, Penn State Milton S. Hershey Medical Center, Hershey, Pennsylvania

MARYN ANNE VALDEZ, MD
PGY-3 Family Medicine Resident, Penn State Hershey Family and Community Medicine Residency Program, Department of Family Medicine, Penn State Milton S. Hershey Medical Center, Hershey, Pennsylvania

ALAN ZAKARIA, DO, MS
Nahed A. Zakaria MD, P.C., Troy, Michigan

Contents

> Acne is a common complaint in the primary care clinics. It has not only physical implications but also psychological. This article discusses the epidemiology, pathophysiology, and criteria for making the diagnosis. It also discusses endocrine disorders that may be the cause of acne. Treatment and management are discussed by subtype. Acne mechanica or sports-related acne is also discussed.

> Urticaria is a common condition that involves pruritic, raised skin wheals. Although urticaria is a benign, self-limiting condition, it may cause frustration for patients, often because of its chronicity and its tendency to recur. It can also be a life-threatening allergic reaction. Diagnosis is made clinically. It affects 20% of the general population. The first-line treatment for non-remitting cases includes H-1anti-histamines. However, other therapies may be employed. Other allergy-mediated skin conditions include angioedema, contact dermatitis, and atopic dermatitis. Diagnosis is clinical, and management focuses on prevention, avoiding triggers, and treating the itching and inflammation that accompany these conditions.

> Skin and soft tissue infections account for 0.5% of outpatient visits to primary care. Skin and soft tissue infections can usually be managed in an outpatient setting. However, there are certain circumstances as discussed in this article that require more urgent care or inpatient management. Primary care providers should be able to diagnose, manage, and provide appropriate follow-up care for these frequently seen skin infections. This article provides family physicians with a comprehensive review of the assessment and management of common bacterial skin infections.

> Superficial fungal infections grow in dark and moist areas and invade various parts of the body. These infections are easily treatable in

immunocompetent individuals. In immunosuppressed individuals, the presentation can be quite severe, requiring use of more potent antifungal agents. The treatment for these conditions consists of topical antifungal agents, creams, and oral systemic medications. The use of prednisone can alter the appearance of superficial fungal infections, making them difficult to diagnose. It is important for primary care providers to become adept at understanding the epidemiology, transmission, clinical presentation, diagnosis techniques, and treatment options available.

In the vast world of skin diseases, viral skin disorders account for a significant percentage. Most viral skin diseases present with an exanthem (skin rash) and, oftentimes, an accompanying enanthem (lesions involving the mucosal membrane). In this article, the various viral skin diseases are explored, including viral childhood exanthems (measles, rubella, erythema infectiosum, and roseola), herpes viruses (herpes simplex virus, varicella zoster virus, Kaposi sarcoma herpes virus, viral zoonotic infections [orf, monkeypox, ebola, smallpox]), and several other viral skin diseases, such as human papilloma virus, hand, foot, and mouth disease, molluscum contagiosum, and Gianotti-Crosti syndrome.

Alopecias represent a heterogeneous group of disorders with different etiologies, presentations, and treatment options. The evaluation of the hair loss patient includes a comprehensive clinical history and physical examination; appropriate laboratory testing; and if indicated, a scalp biopsy. Treatment methods vary depending on the type of alopecia and include watchful waiting, topical and systemic formulations, surgery, and treatment of any underlying or associated conditions. Referral to a dermatologist is helpful in diagnostically challenging and difficult-to-treat cases. Alopecia can cause emotional, mental, and social distress to patients. Early diagnosis and timely institution of appropriate treatment are helpful and comforting to those affected by this disease.

Sunburn, thermal, and chemical injuries to the skin are common in the United States and worldwide. Initial management is determined by type and extent of injury with special care to early management of airway, breathing, and circulation. Fluid management has typically been guided by the Parkland formula, whereas some experts now question this. Each type of skin injury has its own pathophysiology and resultant complications. All primary care physicians should have at least a basic knowledge of management of acute and chronic skin injuries.

Dermatologic complaints are encountered frequently by the primary care provider. Patients often are required as well as want to see their primary care provider before referral to a specialist. Therefore, primary care providers must be skilled in a variety of topics including dermatology. Certain dermatologic manifestations are associated with, or indicative of, systemic diseases. Primary care providers must be knowledgeable in diagnosis, evaluation, and treatment of dermatologic conditions, as well as when to appropriately refer. This article reviews common dermatologic manifestations of systemic diseases.

Pressure and friction injuries are common throughout the lifespan. A detailed history of the onset and progression of friction and pressure injuries is key to aiding clinicians in determining the underlying mechanism behind the development of the injury. Modifying or removing the forces that are creating pressure or friction is the key to both prevention and healing of these injuries. Proper care of pressure and friction injuries to the skin is important to prevent the development of infection. Patient education on positioning and ergonomics can help to prevent recurrence of pressure and friction injuries.

Skin cancer accounts for most malignancies across the globe. They are primarily divided into melanoma and nonmelanoma skin malignancies. Nonmelanoma skin cancer includes basal cell carcinoma and squamous cell carcinoma. Fair skin and chronic ultraviolet B exposure are the most important risk factors. Primary prevention is achieved by avoiding sun exposure and tanning beds.

The two epidermal parasitic skin infections most commonly encountered by primary care physicians in developed countries are scabies and pediculosis. Pediculosis can be further subdivided into pediculosis capitis, corporis, and pubis. This article presents a summary of information and a review of the literature on clinical findings, diagnosis, and treatment of these commonly encountered parasitic skin infestations.

A variety of nail deformities commonly presents in the primary care office. An understanding of nail anatomy coupled with inspection of the nails at routine office visits can reveal undetected disorders. Some problems are benign, and treatment should be attempted by the primary care provider, such as onychomycosis, paronychia, or ingrown toenails. For conditions such as benign melanonychia, longitudinal ridges, isolated Beau lines, and onycholysis, clinicians may offer reassurance to patients who are concerned about the change in their nails. For deformities such as early pterygium or clubbing, a thorough evaluation and referral to an appropriate specialist may be warranted.

PRIMARY CARE:
CLINICS IN OFFICE PRACTICE

RELATED INTEREST

Medical Clinics, November 2015 (Vol. 99, Issue 6)
Dermatology
Roy M. Colven, *Editor*
Available at: http://www.medical.theclinics.com/

THE CLINICS ARE AVAILABLE ONLINE!
Access your subscription at:
www.theclinics.com

Foreword

Pattern Recognition

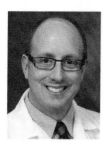

Joel J. Heidelbaugh, MD, FAAFP, FACG
Consulting Editor

I unfortunately remember getting only very cursory dermatology teaching in medical school relative to actual patients: "If it's wet, keep it dry. If it's dry, keep it wet. Try some steroid ointment. And when in doubt, biopsy it." Obviously, dermatology is far more complicated than these 4 very superficial pearls. In daily practice, my colleagues and I agree that to gain expertise in dermatology, clinicians require lots and lots of repetition, a keen sense of pattern recognition, and the willingness to ask a colleague for their opinion! I can't make it through a day of clinic without seeing a patient for a dermatologic complaint. The visit usually begins with a request for the patient to be referred to dermatology, likely assuming that only a dermatologist can manage their concern. Most patients are very pleased to learn that their primary care clinician can handle their needs.

Similar to most other organ-system-based disorders, the statistics for dermatologic conditions are often very frightening:

- An estimated 73,870 new cases of invasive melanoma will be diagnosed in the United States in 2015, and an estimated 9940 people will die of melanoma in 2015.[1]
- More than 419,000 cases of skin cancer in the United States each year are linked to indoor tanning, including about 245,000 basal cell carcinomas, 168,000 squamous cell carcinomas, and 6200 melanomas.[2]
- An estimated 1957 indoor tanners landed in US emergency rooms in 2012 after burning their skin or eyes, fainting, or suffering other injuries.[3]

This issue of *Primary Care: Clinics in Office Practice* is dedicated to dermatologic conditions commonly encountered in primary care practices. Topics presented in detail include acne; urticarial, bacterial, viral, parasitic, and fungal infections; skin cancers; nail deformities; and the very challenging dermatologic manifestations of systemic diseases. Dr George Pujalte and his colleagues deserve praise for their detailed review of the literature on these topics as well as their effort in presenting

http://dx.doi.org/10.1016/j.pop.2015.09.002
0095-4543/15/$ – see front matter © 2015 Published by Elsevier Inc.
primarycare.theclinics.com

this material in a logical and useful fashion for primary care clinicians. We hope that our readers will use this reference in their daily practices, augment their skills, and improve the outcomes of their patients' dermatologic conditions.

Joel J. Heidelbaugh, MD, FAAFP, FACG
Departments of Family Medicine and Urology
University of Michigan Medical School
Ann Arbor, MI 48109, USA

Ypsilanti Health Center
200 Arnet Suite 200
Ypsilanti, MI 48198, USA

E-mail address:
jheidel@umich.edu

REFERENCES

1. American Cancer Society. Cancer facts and figures 2015. Available at: http://www.cancer.org/acs/groups/content/@editorial/documents/document/acspc-044552.pdf. Accessed August 27, 2015.
2. Wehner M, Chren M-M, Nameth D, et al. International prevalence of indoor tanning: a systematic review and meta-analysis. JAMA Dermatol 2014;150(4):390–400.
3. Guy GP Jr, Watson M, Haileyesus T, et al. Indoor tanning-related injuries treated in a national sample of US hospital emergency departments. JAMA Intern Med 2015; 175(2):309–11.

Preface

Beyond Superficial: Primary Care Dermatology

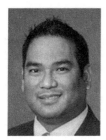

George G.A. Pujalte, MD, FACSM
Editor

This issue is written for primary care physicians, who are often the first to see skin conditions in their clinics. Skin conditions are often not stand-alone ailments; they may be the result of underlying conditions that may worsen if not diagnosed early. It is the responsibility of primary care physicians to recognize skin manifestations of such conditions. Some conditions are also uniquely linked to certain segments of the population, such as athletes or women. The implications of skin conditions in sports medicine also need to be known to primary care physicians.

This issue aims to address all manner of ways skin conditions may present in primary care clinics and on the first visit. It discusses the tests that need to be ordered and addresses the latest, evidence-based treatments for each ailment. Naturally, images and figures are used extensively in this issue, and it is hoped that they serve the primary care clinician well as a quick resource in a busy clinic.

Comprising the collective expertise of experienced primary care physicians and dermatologists alike, this issue is an amalgamation of knowledge. It is an accumulation of the insight of physicians who see skin conditions early in their progression, as well as a range of patients and conditions that go beyond dermatology, and the invaluable input of learned dermatologists, sharing their knowledge borne of specialized treatment of skin diseases. Gathering images that would prove useful to potential readers proved to be a challenging undertaking, as was the difficult process of coordinating input from physician authors from different institutions. In the end, however, we hope this issue becomes a testament to the benefits of working together and sharing knowledge.

I am thankful to my colleagues from and at the University of the Philippines, the Mount Sinai Hospital in Chicago, the University of Michigan, Penn State University, the Mayo Clinic, and other institutions, for their efforts and their willingness to push through with this project despite the challenges posed by distance and individual schedules. Without them, this issue would not have been possible.

Prim Care Clin Office Pract 42 (2015) xv–xvi
http://dx.doi.org/10.1016/j.pop.2015.09.001
0095-4543/15/$ – see front matter © 2015 Published by Elsevier Inc.

primarycare.theclinics.com

The most rewarding way to read this issue, in my opinion, is to peruse the images as delineated by the text and the headings. Once a condition seen in clinics appears compatible, more details can be read. In instances where images are not available, the descriptions of the skin conditions may be used; we have endeavored to make the descriptions as useful as possible in this regard. We hope that each article in the issue provides ample guidance for every skin condition of interest to primary care physicians.

George G.A. Pujalte, MD, FACSM
Family Medicine and Sports Medicine
Department of Family Medicine
Mayo Clinic
4500 San Pablo Road
Jacksonville, FL 32224, USA

E-mail address:
pujalte.george@mayo.edu

Evaluation and Management of Acne

Paul A. Botros, MD[a],*, Gary Tsai, MD[a], George G.A. Pujalte, MD[b]

KEYWORDS

- Acne • Evaluation • Management • Treatment • Retinoid • Sports medicine

KEY POINTS

- Acne vulgaris is a common disorder of the pilosebaceous follicles that affects adolescents and can persist into adulthood.
- The psychological and economic impact is significant and may prove challenging to address in the clinical setting.
- The diagnosis of acne vulgaris can be made from the patient's history and physical examination and can be effectively treated in the primary care setting.

INTRODUCTION

Acne vulgaris, commonly known as acne, is the most common skin condition affecting up to 95% of adolescents and young adults in the United States.[1,2] It typically begins at puberty. It is estimated that acne affects 9.4% of the global population.[3] Clinical presentations can vary drastically among patients, with mild to severe disease. Patients, particularly adolescents, may therefore experience significant social and emotional symptoms of embarrassment with associated psychological symptoms of depression or anxiety that affect social lives.[4] Fortunately, there are several acne treatments available,[1] but diagnosis and treatment guidelines are lacking and variations exist across specialties.[4] This article reviews the epidemiology and pathophysiology and also discusses how primary care clinicians can appropriately diagnose patients with acne.

EPIDEMIOLOGY

Acne usually begins at puberty and affects adolescents of both genders. It is most common at ages 12 to 25 years.[5] More than 85% of teenagers experience some

Disclosure Statement: The authors have nothing to disclose.
a Department of Family and Community Medicine, Penn State Milton S. Hershey Medical Center, Hershey, PA 17033, USA; b Family Medicine and Sports Medicine, Department of Family Medicine, Mayo Clinic, 4500 San Pablo Road, Jacksonville, FL 32224, USA
* Corresponding author. 736 Ferris Way, Hershey, PA 17033.
E-mail address: PBOTROS@HMC.PSU.EDU

form of acne.[6] Although acne tends to resolve before the age of 30 years, it may persist into adulthood. Prevalence studies in adults 20 years or older have shown that women were being affected at higher rates than men.[6] It is a chronic disease that can persist for many years. There is limited amount of research about what specific factors predict whether it will last into adulthood.[7]

PATHOPHYSIOLOGY

Acne vulgaris is a disease of pilosebaceous follicles.[7] Studies indicate that pathogenesis of acne involves 4 main processes:

1. Androgen-induced increase in sebum production, usually around puberty
2. Altered keratinization of the sebaceous duct, leading to comedone formation
3. Inflammation around the sebaceous gland
4. Bacterial colonization of hair follicles on the face, neck, chest, and back by *Propionibacterium acnes*.[7]

Current therapies target these 4 factors for acute control of flare-ups and long-term maintenance.[8] The sequence of events and how these factors interact remain unclear, but there are various underlying causes of these changes. Increased androgen production leads to abnormal epithelial desquamation and follicular obstruction, which leads to the formation of the microcomedone, the precursor lesion in acne.[9] Studies have shown that immune changes and inflammation may stimulate pilosebaceous vasculature before keratinization, which is led by CD4[+] lymphocytes and macrophages. It has been hypothesized that interleukin (IL) 1a induces cytokines to activate local endothelial cells, which in turn upregulate inflammatory vascular makers such as E-selectin, vascular cell adhesion molecule 1, intercellular adhesion molecule 1, and HLA-DR around pilosebaceous follicles. This is due to a linoleic acid deficiency caused by excess sebum and agitation of barrier function within the follicle.[10,11]

Comedones form as a result of increased cell division and cohesion of cells lining the follicular lumen. When cells accumulate abnormally, mix with sebum, and partially obstruct the follicular opening, they form a closed comedone, or whitehead. If the follicular opening is larger, keratin buildup becomes more visible and may darken to form an open comedone, or blackhead. *Propionibacterium acnes* colonizes different pilosebaceous units and leads to inflammation via the production of inflammatory mediators, activating toll-like receptor-2, which results in the production of proinflammatory cytokines such as IL-12 and IL-8, leading to the formation of inflammatory papules and pustules.[4,12] Improved understanding of acne development suggests that acne is a disease consisting of a combination of the innate and adaptive immune systems, as well as inflammatory events. Treatment, therefore, targets both immune system activation and inflammatory pathways.[10]

DIAGNOSIS

Acne is diagnosed by the identification of lesions on the skin on physical examination.[5] However, before initiating treatment, it is important to assess and evaluate a patient by obtaining a standard history of present illness and review medications and prescriptions that the patient has been taking. Any hormonal influences caused by medications may affect natural hormonal processes, leading to possible acne. The patient should be assessed by asking about the duration of symptoms, locations on the body, variations of weather exposure, and stressors. In addition, any information regarding current treatments for acne and failures may be helpful in guiding treatment.

Additional information to obtain from women includes information about flare-ups that may occur with menstruation, menstruation history, pregnancy history, oral contraceptives, and cosmetics. Furthermore, family history regarding endocrine abnormalities, acne, polycystic ovarian syndrome, and skin disorders may also be important to evaluate.

On physical examination, useful clinical categorization of acne is based on predominate morphology: noninflammatory open or closed comedones (blackheads and whiteheads) to inflammatory lesions consisting of erythematous papules, pustules, or cystlike nodules.[4]

Severity can be classified as mild, moderate, or severe depending on the number of comedones or inflammatory lesions (**Table 1**).

There are many other conditions that can mimic acne, some of which contain the term acne in their nomenclature, but they lack the presence of comedones. Differential diagnoses include the following[13]:

- Keratosis pilaris
- Malaria
- Milia
- Rosacea
- Periorificial dermatitis
- Molluscum contagiosum
- Flat warts
- Infection
- Acne venenata
- Bilateral nevus comedonicus
- Tuberous sclerosis
- Demodicidosis
- Reaction to medication (corticosteroid, dactinomycin, lithium, phenytoin)

Table 1
Types and severity classifications of acne

Types of Acne	
Comedonal (noninflammatory)	Dilated hair follicles filled with keratin, sebum, and bacteria Whitehead: closed comedone Blackhead: open comedone with darkened mass of skin debris
Papulopustular (inflammatory)	Papule: pink/red inflammatory lesions 2–5 mm in diameter Pustule: superficial papules with visible core of purulent material
Nodular (inflammatory) nodule	Solid, raised inflammatory lesions >5 mm in diameter
Severity classifications	
Mild	<20 comedones or <15 inflammatory lesions or <30 lesions total
Moderate	20–100 comedones or 15–50 inflammatory lesions or 30–125 lesions total
Severe	>5 nodules or >50 total inflammatory lesions or >125 lesions total

Data from Liao DC. Management of acne. J Family Practice 2003;52(1):43–51; and Krakowski AC, Stendardo S, Eichenfield LF. Practical considerations in acne treatment and the clinical impact of topical combination therapy. Pediatr Dermatol 2008;25(Suppl 1):1–14.

- Pseudofolliculitis barbae
- In prepubertal children, consider
  - Cushing syndrome
  - Congenital adrenal hyperplasia
  - Premature adrenarche
  - Polycystic ovarian syndrome
  - Gonadal, adrenal, or ovarian tumor
  - Precocious puberty

Routine endocrinologic testing for androgen excess is not typically indicated but may have use for children who have signs of androgen excess (eg, body odor, axillary/pubic hair, infrequent menses, hirsutism).[14]

Acne lesions may vary widely and range from noninflammatory open or closed comedones to inflammatory lesions, which may include papules, pustules, or nodules. They are likely to occur on the face, neck, chest, and back, where sebaceous glands are more concentrated. Nodular acne is characterized by a predominance of large inflammatory nodules or pseudocysts and is often accompanied by scarring or the presence of sinus tracts when adjacent nodules coalesce.[4]

TREATMENT

There is no universal classification system for acne vulgaris because of the wide variety of presentations of the disease. Reduction in existing microcomedones and prevention of the formation of new ones is central to the management of all acne lesions.[4] Treatment that targets both immune system activation and inflammatory pathways is, therefore, desirable.

MANAGEMENT OF ACNE

There are multiple modalities for the management of acne. Treatments are focused on several factors including

1. Normalization of keratin cells and sebum production to prevent pore blockage
2. Microbicidal activity
3. Hormonal therapy

Table 2 summarizes the treatment of acne by type.

Before any pharmacologic intervention, the patient should be counseled regarding overscrubbing of the skin, as this behavior may dry and irritate the skin, thereby worsening acne. The patient should also be counseled against squeezing or picking comedones, as this promotes scar formation. Patients with acne should also be screened for depression as they are often disturbed by their body image.[17]

TOPICAL RETINOIDS

Topical retinoids are vitamin A analogs that normalize keratinization, which then leads to a reduction of follicular occlusion.[13] In addition to treating active acne, retinoids may improve resolution of acne-related skin hyperpigmentation.[15] They are used for the treatment of both noninflammatory and inflammatory acne and should be used as first-line treatments. They are considered the mainstay for maintenance therapy.

Patients should be counseled on evening applications, as retinoids are associated with sun sensitivity. Patients should also be counseled that they should apply small amounts of the medication and gradually increase until reaching the amount prescribed, as these cause irritation, dry skin, erythema, and flaking.

Table 2
Methods of acne treatment by type

Mild Acne	
Comedonal	Mild Papular/Pustular
First line: topical retinoid	First line: topical retinoid and topical antimicrobial
Alternatives: topical retinoid or azelaic acid or salicylic acid	Alternatives: topical retinoid or azelaic acid or salicylic acid
Alternatives: none	Alternatives: none
Maintenance: topical retinoid	Maintenance: topical retinoid
Moderate Acne	
Moderate Papular/Pustular	Nodular
First line: oral antibiotics and topical retinoid; may also consider the addition of benzoyl peroxide	First line: oral isotretinoin and topical retinoid; may also consider the addition of benzoyl peroxide and azelaic acid
Alternatives: topical retinoid or azelaic acid or salicylic acid	Oral isotretinoin or alternative oral antibiotic with a topical retinoid and benzoyl peroxide or azelaic acid
Alternatives for women: oral antiandrogen and a topical retinoid or azelaic acid, with or without an antimicrobial	Alternatives: oral antiandrogen with a topical retinoid with or without an oral antibiotic and with or without an alternative antimicrobial
Maintenance: topical retinoid	Maintenance: topical retinoid with or without benzoyl peroxide
Severe Acne	
Nodular/Conglobate	
First line: oral isotretinoin	
Alternatives: high-dose oral antibiotic with a topical retinoid and benzoyl peroxide	
Alternatives for women: high-dose oral antiandrogen with a topical retinoid, with or without a topical antimicrobial	
Maintenance: topical retinoid with or without a benzoyl peroxide	

Data from Refs.[9,13–16]

TOPICAL ANTIMICROBIALS

Topical antimicrobials decrease proinflammatory bacteria such as *P acnes*. The most commonly used topical antimicrobial is benzyl peroxide. Other examples include erythromycin, clindamycin, sulfacetamide, and dapsone. Azelaic acid is a topical antimicrobial that naturally has mild anti-inflammatory properties that may help with acne-induced postinflammatory hyperpigmentation. Topical antimicrobials are generally prescribed in conjunction with topical retinoids.[14] Similar to retinoids, topical antimicrobials may cause skin irritation or dry skin.

ORAL ANTIBIOTICS

The use of oral antibiotics should be limited to inflammatory acne and acne that involves the chest or back. Oral antibiotics are not indicated for long-term use. They are indicated in those with acne involving the chest or the back.[9,14] When prescribed, they should be used in conjunction with topical retinoids. Oral antibiotics should be used only for short courses as they contribute to *P acnes* antibiotic resistance and only when absolutely necessary. Examples of commonly used antibiotics include macrolides, such as erythromycin, or tetracyclines, such as minocycline. Minocycline is most commonly prescribed as it induces more rapid improvement in inflammatory acne than tetracycline.[16] Many oral antibiotics are also associated with photosensitivity.[16]

HORMONAL THERAPY AND ORAL CONTRACEPTIVES

Patients who benefit from hormonal therapy are divided into 2 categories: (1) women with acne related to menses and (2) women with hyperandrogenism. The former may be treated with combined oral contraceptives that are approved by the US Food and Drug Administration for use in acne.[18] Progestin-only pills may worsen acne. Women with hyperandrogenism may benefit from androgen-reducing medications and/or androgen receptor blockers. However, extreme caution should be used with these medications because of possible feminizing effects on a developing fetus.[18]

ORAL RETINOIDS

Oral retinoids work by normalizing keratinization of cells, similar to topical retinoids. They have also been shown to induce apoptosis of sebaceous gland cells.[19]

Oral retinoids are effective for the treatment of severe, nodular acne. They may be used as monotherapy, under careful supervision. Only authorized physicians can prescribe oral retinoids. Women must be on active birth control when given oral retinoids, because of teratogenicity.[9,13,18] Oral retinoids have also been linked to ulcerative colitis, depression, and suicidal ideation.[19] These symptoms can also be associated with pseudotumor cerebri and hypervitaminosis A.[19]

TREATMENT OF ACNE MECHANICA (SPORTS-INDUCED ACNE)

Acne mechancia is acne that is associated with athletes and is triggered by heat, friction, or pressure. It can occur anywhere on the body. It can appear as papules or pustules. Most cases respond well to topical benzyl peroxide and salicylic acid, along with improved hygiene.[20]

SUMMARY

Acne vulgaris is a common disorder of the pilosebaceous follicles that affects adolescents and can persist into adulthood. The psychological and economic impact is significant and may prove challenging to address in the clinical setting. The diagnosis of acne vulgaris can be made from the patient's history and physical examination. It can be effectively treated in the primary care setting.

REFERENCES

1. American Academy of Dermatology. Available at: https://www.aad.org/dermatology-a-to-z/diseases-and-treatments/a--d/acne. Accessed April 10, 2015.
2. Zouboulis CC, Bettoli V. Management of severe acne. Br J Dermatol 2015; 172(Suppl 1):27–36.
3. Tan JK, Bhate K. A global perspective on the epidemiology of acne. Br J Dermatol 2015;172(Suppl 1):3–12.
4. Eichenfield LF, Krakowski AC, Piggott C, et al. Evidence-based recommendations for the diagnosis and treatment of pediatric acne. Pediatrics 2013; 131(Suppl 3):S163–86.

5. White GM. Recent findings in the epidemiologic evidence, classification, and subtypes of acne vulgaris. J Am Acad Dermatol 1998;39(2 Pt 3):S34–7.
6. Collier CN, Harper JC, Cafardi JA, et al. The prevalence of acne in adults 20 years and older. J Am Acad Dermatol 2008;58(1):56–9.
7. Williams HC, Dellavalle RP, Garner S. Acne vulgaris. Lancet 2012;379(9813): 361–72.
8. Titus S, Hodge J. Diagnosis and treatment of acne. Am Fam Physician 2012; 86(8):734–40.
9. Dawson AL, Dellavalle RP. Acne vulgaris. BMJ 2013;346:f2634.
10. Thiboutot D, Gollnick H, Bettoli V, et al. New insides into the management of acne: an update from the global alliance to improve outcomes in acne group. J Am Acad Dermatol 2009;60:S1–50.
11. Jeremy AH, Holland DB, Roberts SG, et al. Inflammatory events are involved in acne lesion initiation. J Invest Dermatol 2003;121(1):20–7.
12. Tanghetti EA. The role of inflammation in the pathology of acne. J Clin Aesthet Dermatol 2013;6(9):27–35.
13. Whitney KM, Ditre CM. Management strategies for acne vulgaris. Clin Cosmet Investig Dermatol 2011;4:41–53.
14. Strauss JS, Krowchuk DP, Leyden JJ, et al. Guidelines of care for acne vulgaris management. J Am Acad Dermatol 2007;56(4):651–63.
15. Chandrashekhar BS, Anitha M, Ruparelia M, et al. Tretinoin nanogel 0.025% versus conventional gel 0.025% in patients with acne vulgaris: a randomized, active controlled, multicentre, parallel group, phase IV clinical trial. J Clin Diagn Res 2015;9(1):WC04–9.
16. Leyden JJ, Del Rosso JQ. Oral antibiotic therapy for acne vulgaris: pharmacokinetic and pharmacodynamic perspectives. J Clin Aesthet Dermatol 2011; 4(2):40–7.
17. Bowe WP, Doyle AK, Crerand CE, et al. Body image disturbance in patients with acne vulgaris. J Clin Aesthet Dermatol 2011;4(7):35–41.
18. Ebede TL, Arch EL, Berson D. Hormonal treatment of acne in women. J Clin Aesthet Dermatol 2009;2(12):16–22.
19. Gollnick HP, Zouboulis CC. Not all acne is acne vulgaris. Dtsch Arztebl Int 2014; 111(17):301–12.
20. Emer J, Sivek R, Marciniak B. Sports dermatology: part 1 of 2. Traumatic or mechanical injuries, inflammatory conditions, and exacerbations of pre-existing conditions. J Clin Aesthet Dermatol 2015;8(4):31–43.

Urticaria and Allergy-Mediated Conditions

 CrossMark

Lena Jafilan, MD[a], Charis James, MD, MPH[b],*

KEYWORDS

- Allergy • Antihistamines • Hives • Swelling • Urticaria • Angioedema

KEY POINTS

- Urticaria is a common condition that involves pruritic, raised skin wheals, which may or may not be edematous.
- Although urticaria is a benign, self-limiting condition, it may cause frustration for patients often because of its chronicity and its tendency to recur. It can also be a life-threatening allergic reaction, and it affects 20% of the general population.
- The first-line treatment for nonremitting cases consists of H-1anti-histamines.
- Other allergy-mediated skin conditions include angioedema, contact dermatitis, and atopic dermatitis; allergy-mediated conditions affect a broad range of the population.
- Diagnosis is clinical, and management focuses on prevention, avoiding triggers, and treating the itching and inflammation that accompany these conditions.

DESCRIPTION

Urticarial rashes are characterized by the sudden eruption of wheals of various shapes and sizes. The lesions are described as erythematous papules or plaques that may be blanchable. Their sizes can vary from a few millimeters to several centimeters. They are frequently pruritic or burn, eventually resolving within a few days, with no residual skin changes. Lesions lasting for more than 6 weeks are considered chronic urticaria.

Urticaria results from a cascade involving immunologic events. It begins with the degranulation of mast cells, which is a stimulus for the release of other cell mediators. These mediators include histamine, bradykinin, leukotrienes, prostaglandins, and other vasodilatory substances. In turn, these cause plasma cell extravasation into the dermis, resulting in the characteristic raised, pruritic, edematous urticarial lesions.[1]

Urticaria may or may not present with angioedema. Angioedema is inflammation of the lips, face, upper airway, and/or extremities. Although urticaria and angioedema

[a] Penn State Milton S. Hershey Medical Center, Department of Family and Community Medicine, 566 Dickens Drive, Hummelstown, Hershey, PA 17036, USA; [b] Penn State Milton S. Hershey Medical Center, Department of Family and Community Medicine, 114 Stonebrook Drive, Palmyra, Hershey, PA 17078, USA
* Corresponding author.
E-mail address: cjames3@hmc.psu.edu

Prim Care Clin Office Pract 42 (2015) 473–483
http://dx.doi.org/10.1016/j.pop.2015.08.002
0095-4543/15/$ – see front matter Published by Elsevier Inc.

primarycare.theclinics.com

may have similar underlying physiologic cell-mediator mechanisms, the actual skin locations will vary. Angioedema presents in the deeper dermis and subcutaneous tissues, whereas urticaria involves superficial dermis.

In immunoglobulin E (IgE)-mediated reactions, a type 1 cell-type reaction is the main proposed mechanism (**Fig. 1**). This is seen in allergic reactions that take place within minutes to hours after allergen exposure. A well-studied example of IgE- and mast cell-mediated urticaria is cold urticaria. In affected people, an extremity immersed in an ice bath precipitates angioedema of the distal portion, with urticaria appearing within minutes of the challenge. Marked mast cell degranulation is seen histologically, with associated edema of underlying skin structures and elevated levels of histamine arising in the affected extremity compared with the unaffected extremity. Similar events were also demonstrated in the biopsy-proven mast cell degranulation associated with attacks of cholinergic urticaria and exercise-induced urticaria.[2]

For the most part, triggers may be identified in acute cases, but a specific trigger may only be found in 10% to 20% of chronic cases.[2]

Common acute urticarial causes include food, insects, medications, and infections. Infections make up over 80% of acute pediatric cases.[2] Although common viral, bacterial, and parasitic infections can be identifiable, the pathogenesis for these as

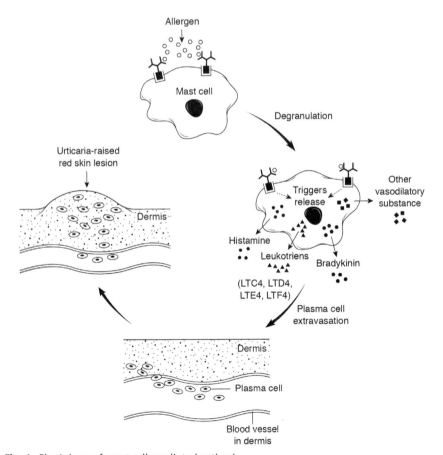

Fig. 1. Physiology of mast cell-mediated urticaria.

causes of urticaria remains unclear. Clinicians should be aware that acute cases may even be an initial sign in pediatric patients with human immunodeficiency virus (HIV).[2]

EPIDEMIOLOGY

Family practitioners should be well-versed in the approach to patients presenting with urticaria. With the lifetime prevalence of about 20% in adults aged 20 to 40 years old, hospital admissions for severe forms could be prevented solely by greater clinician knowledge.[3]

Incidence

Urticaria occurs in all ages. The acute form is more commonly seen in the pediatric population. The more chronic form is seen mainly in adults. More males are affected compared to females.[3]

Prevalence

Among the general population, 15% to 25% are affected by this condition. Causes of acute urticaria include infection (49%), drugs (5%), and food allergies (3%). Chronic urticaria is less common, only seen about 3% of the time.[2]

DIAGNOSIS

The diagnosis of urticaria is essentially clinical. However, ancillary tests to determine the etiology can sometimes be employed. Although typically a benign, self-limiting condition, urticaria may contribute to one's impairment in performing daily functions.

The patient may describe the sudden appearance of raised lesions or wheals of varying shapes and sizes, presenting virtually anywhere on the body (**Figs. 2** and **3**). The lesions are usually described as intensely pruritic. The lesions may also be described as stinging, giving a pins and needles sensation, or even painful. In acute urticaria, the lesions usually disappear in less than 24 hours, lasting less than 6 weeks. Chronic urticaria by definition lasts more than 6 weeks. It is important to try and tease out the inciting exposure via a thorough review of the exposures to foods, medication, cosmetics, chemicals, or environmental factors.

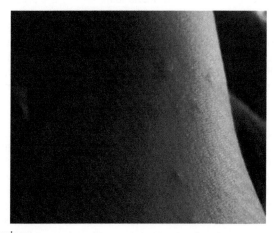

Fig. 2. Urticaria lesions.

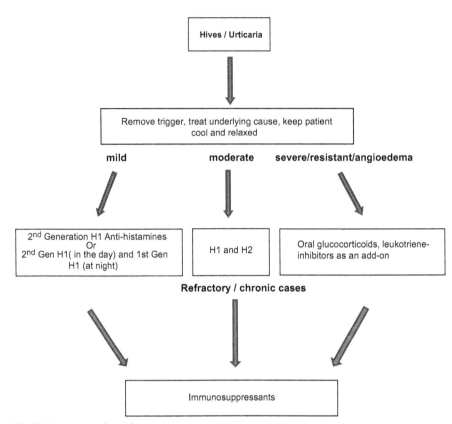

Fig. 3. Treatment algorithm.

On physical examination, the lesions can range in size from a few millimeters to several centimeters in size. The lesions can be sharply demarcated, shaped irregularly, round, oval, rhomboid, serpiginous, or linear. The size and shapes are transient and may change over time (see **Fig. 2**).

Tests are usually employed when urticaria lasts for more than 24 hours. A biopsy can be done to rule out urticarial vasculitis. In chronic urticaria, a complete blood cell count (CBC) with differential, erythrocyte sedimentation rate (ESR), *Helicobacter pylori* testing, and thyroid function tests may be helpful to rule out underlying disorders. For cold-induced urticaria, testing for cryoglobulins and hepatitis testing will be helpful. In addition, allergy skin testing may be useful to determine the underlying cause in acute urticaria. Clinical patterns may be helpful for diagnosis of urticaria (**Table 1**).

Causes

About 50% of urticaria is idiopathic.[4] The causes that can be identified are several, varied, and usually found in acute urticaria. Mast cell degranulation is the underlying mechanism that triggers urticaria. Histamine is released, causing vasodilation. Vasodilation leads to the shifting of fluid to go outside the blood vessels, resulting in localized edema. Some of the more common causes include infections and allergic reactions. Infections can be viral, bacterial, or parasitic. The allergic reactions can be caused by food, insects, medications, chemicals, physical stimuli, and

Table 1
Clinical patterns in the diagnosis of urticaria

Clinical Pattern	Probable Diagnosis
Gastrointestinal upset, respiratory distress, autonomic dysfunction	Anaphylaxis
Food exposure	Food allergy
Fevers, chills, systemic signs of infection, recent travel	Infection
History of starting new medication	Medication allergy
Stimuli such as strong emotions, stress, exercise	Cholinergic urticaria
Exposure to vibration, pressure, cold	Physical urticaria

environmental triggers. Some medications such as narcotics and antibiotics can directly induce mast cell degranulation, leading to urticarial skin lesions. The causes can be classified as IgE-mediated, bradykinin-mediated, complement-mediated, and nonimmunologic. **Table 2** describes the different classes and give examples for each class.

Treatment

Avoiding triggers is the primary management approach. The patient should be kept relaxed and in a cool environment. Patients should be advised to avoid hot showers, as they can exacerbate pruritus. Most cases of acute urticaria will resolve on their own, and treatment is seldom necessary. It is helpful to reassure the patient of this fact. Treatment is usually employed for chronic disease and focuses mainly on symptom relief. The pruritus related to urticaria is one of the primary foci of therapy. **Table 3** reviews the major classes of drugs and examples from each class that are used to treat urticaria.

Add-on treatments that are sometimes used in resistant cases include leukotriene inhibitors such as montelukast, zafirlukastm, and zileuton. In severe cases, a short course of steroids may be employed with the initiation of antihistamine treatment. Steroids are avoided in chronic urticaria, as poor response is usually seen, and steroids may come with a high risk of toxicity.

For chronic disease and poorly responsive cases, cyclosporine and monoclonal anti-IgE antibodies (omalizumab) may be used. If an underlying disease process such as infection or hypothyroidism is found to be the cause, treatment is indicated.[4] An approach to treatment in summarized in the treatment algorithm found in **Fig. 3**.

Table 2
The different classes of urticaria etiology

Etiologic Class	Examples
Bradykinin-mediated	Angiotensin-converting enzyme (ACE), hereditary angioedema
IgE-mediated	Pollen, food, medications, fungi, molds, parasitic infections, insect venom
Complement-mediated	Necrotizing vasculitis, serum sickness, reactions to blood products
Nonimmune-mediated	Direct mast degranulation agents (narcotic/opiates, muscle relaxants, radiocontrast, vancomycin), nonsteroidal anti-inflammatory drugs, physical stimuli (cold, heat, vibration, pressure)

	Table 3 Drugs used in the treatment of urticaria		
Class of Drug	Second-Generation, H1 Antihistamines, (First-Line; Nonsedating)	First-Generation, H1 Antihistamines	H2-Blockers
Drug	• Loratidine • Cetirizine • Fexofenadine	• Diphenhydramine • Hydroxyzine • Doxepin	• Cimetidine • Ranitidine • Famotidine

ANGIOEDEMA
Description

Angioedema is local tissue swelling as a result of an allergen triggering the leakage of plasma cells into the mucosa or skin. It is specifically called allergic angioedema. Its pathogenesis is the same as urticaria, and it can be seen along with the latter. It is essentially urticaria that occurs in the mucosa and deeper layers of the skin. Angioedema can also be a part of an anaphylactic reaction. This is a separate entity from hereditary angioedema, which is a nonallergic mechanism caused by bradykinin pathway dysfunction.[5]

Epidemiology

The prevalence and incidence of angioedema are high; however, data on specific rates are not available. Angioedema affects persons of all ages. It affects males and females equally. African-Americans are more commonly affected. This skin reaction accounts for a large portion of hospitalizations caused by allergic skin conditions.[5]

Pathogenesis and Causes

As described in the pathophysiology of urticaria, allergic angioedema is caused by the extravasation of fluid between endothelial cells of blood vessels. This occurs when allergen antigens trigger the release of inflammatory mediators via the degranulation of mast cells. This, in turn, activates a cascade, leading to the leaking of plasma from vasculature. The fluid collects in the deep layers of skin or mucosa. Mucosa that are commonly affected include the throat, tongue, and conjunctiva. In the skin, the face, lips, hand, and genitalia are commonly involved.

Common causes of allergic angioedema are the same as urticaria. These include drugs, food, chemicals, and insect bites.[6]

Diagnosis

The diagnosis is clinical. Swelling will appear suddenly, anywhere from a few minutes to over a few hours. It affects areas where there is loose tissue such as the lips, face, mouth, and genitalia (**Fig. 4**). It is unlike other types of edema in that it spares dependent areas like the legs, and the swelling is asymmetric. Angioedema is usually accompanied with signs and symptoms of allergic or anaphylactic reactions. Laboratory tests do not help with diagnosis, but may be employed in identifying an underlying etiology. Imaging may be useful to evaluate internal mucosal swelling that may be life-threatening.

Treatment

Angioedema can be life-threatening, depending on areas involved. In these cases, such as is the case in anaphylaxis, life support measures should be urgently employed

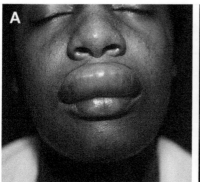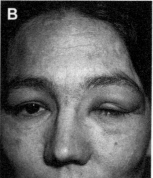

Fig. 4. (*A* and *B*) Swelling of the lip and face caused by angioedema. (*From* [A] Goldstein BG, Goldstein AO. Practical dermatology, edition 2. St Louis: Mosby; 1997; with permission; and [B] James WD, Berger TG, Elston DM. Chapter 6: contact dermatitis and drug eruptions. In: Andrews' diseases of the skin. 12th edition. New York: Elsevier; 2016, with permission.)

to secure airway, breathing, and circulation. Intramuscular epinephrine should be used in anaphylactic cases. Allergic angioedema localized to the skin can be treated with the medications used to treat urticaria (H1/H2 antihistamines or with glucocorticoids) and by removal of inciting allergens.

DERMATITIS
Description

Dermatitis is a skin condition manifested secondary to a trigger substance. Acute or chronic dermatitis may result from chemicals or foreign objects, known as irritant contact dermatitis and allergic contact dermatitis, as the main variants respectively. Although they both are inflammatory skin conditions, irritant contact dermatitis will present by a nonimmune-modulated response, whereas allergic contact dermatitis is a delayed type 4 hypersensitivity immunologic reaction.

Irritant contact dermatitis includes nonimmunologic reaction and dermatitis secondary to foreign irritant that breaks down the epidermal cutaneous layer (chemical or mechanical).

Allergic contact dermatitis includes type 4 delayed hypersensitivity reaction and foreign objects coming into direct contact with skin, resulting in epidermal changes (eg, coins, plants, and fragrances).

Epidemiology

These 2 conditions affect mostly women, with a small percentage of the population genetically predisposed to allergic contact dermatitis.[7–9] A possible suggested reason why women are more affected is that women wear more jewelry than men.

Diagnosis

When a provider encounters a patient presenting with a dermatologic complaint, it is important to get a good history, and ask pertinent information to aid in the proper diagnosis.

Table 4 lists important aspects of history in such cases.

Table 4
Important aspects of history of dermatologic illnesses

History of Present Illness	Signs/Symptoms
• Location and duration	Allergic contact dermatitis
• Size of lesions	• Intensely pruritic rash
• Prurititis	• Papular
• Prior episodes	• Indistinct margins
• Occupational or non-occupational exposure	• Pattern of exposure of allergen
	○ Poison ivy–linear
• New chemicals, including detergents, creams, household cleansers	○ Buttons, earrings–circular (**Fig. 5**)
	Irritant Contact Dermatitis
• Cosmetics: makeup, shampoo, body wash	• Erythema
• Previous treatments and response to treatments	• Fissures
	• Intensely pruritic
• Foreign objects: jewelry, buttons	• Severe cases may present with vesicular lesions or bullae
• New food exposure or preservatives	

Causes

Allergic contact dermatitis and irritant contact dermatitis causes can be classified into 2 categories: occupation exposure and nonoccupational exposure. Similar overlapping areas for both dermatologic states include:

- Healthcare
- Food
- Cosmetology—hair dyes, makeup, creams
- Factory employee—machines, seamstress, metals
- Animals
- Plants—poison ivy, poison oak

Allergic contact dermatitis can also result from nonoccupational exposure to jewelry.

Treatment

Although both dermatologic conditions vary physiologically, they have an overlap in signs and symptoms, and treatment is similar, with a few exceptions (**Tables 5** and **6**).

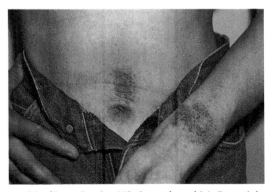

Fig. 5. Contact dermatitis. (*From* Frazier MS, Drzymkowski J. Essentials of human diseases and conditions. 5th edition. New York: Elsevier Saunders; 2012; with permission.)

Table 5
Allergic contact dermatitis

Mild	Moderate/Severe
• Avoid precipitating agent • Medium to high-potency topical steroids (triamcinolone, clobetasol) • Avoid high-potency steroids on the face and flexor surfaces • Topical emollients to form protective barrier • Cool compresses or oatmeal baths	• Systemic corticosteroids • If plant-derived etiology, avoid rebound dermatitis by using 2–3 wk of oral corticosteroids

ECZEMA/ATOPIC DERMATITIS
Description

Atopic dermatitis, frequently called eczema, is a chronic, pruritic skin condition associated with allergies and allergic/atopic conditions such as allergic rhinitis and asthma. Pruritus is a frequently a prominent symptom.

Epidemiology

Most patients are children; approximately 1% to 22% of children are affected. A fair percentage of adults are affected, but 66% had onset of symptoms prior to the age of 7.[10]

Diagnosis

Diagnosis is clinical and based on the following signs and symptoms seen in **Table 7**. Atopic dermatitis can be classified as mild, moderate, or severe based on the extent of symptoms and effects on quality of life. The rash ranges from dry skin to erythematic papules and plaques all the way to thickened, scaly, hyperpigmented skin. Examples of atopic dermatitis can be seen in **Fig. 6**. **Table 7** reviews the clinical classification of atopic dermatitis, based on symptom severity.

These symptoms are frequently associated with a chronic, relapsing, remitting course. Patients usually have a family history of allergies, asthma, or eczema; onset is usually in childhood. The distribution of the rash is usually indicative of a diagnosis. In children, the extensor surfaces of the upper and lower extremities are affected. However, flexural regions such as the antecubital fossa, popliteal fossa, neck, and wrists are more frequently affected in adults (see **Fig. 6**A). Adults with a more extensoral distribution experience poor outcomes.

Treatment

Treatment is aimed at prevention and reducing symptoms. Symptoms that are treated include itching and inflammatory changes of skin (**Table 8**).

Table 6
Irritant contact dermatitis

Mild	Moderate/Severe
• Avoid precipitating agents • Topical emollients to form protective barrier	• Medium- to high-potency topical steroids (triamcinolone, clobetasol) • Systemic corticosteroids are generally not helpful

Table 7
Classification of atopic dermatitis

Classification	Mild	Moderate	Severe
Presentation	+ Dry skin	++ Dry skin	+++ Dry skin
	+/– Mild erythema	+ Erythema	++ Erythema
	+ Pruritus	+/– Excoriation	++ Excoriation
	Little to no impact on quality of life	+ Skin thickening	++ Skin thickening
		++ Pruritus (regular)	Bleeding
		Negative impact on quality of life	Cracking
			Discharge
			Discoloration of skin
			+++ Pruritus (chronic)
			Significant negative impact on quality of life

+ symbol suggests how common symptoms seen.

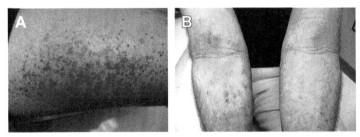

Fig. 6. Atopic dermatitis. (*A*) erythematous eczematous papules, several excoriated, over the left medial thigh. (*B*) Pruritic, dry, scaly, ill-defined patches symmetrically distributed in the bilateral antecubital fossae. (*From* Brinster NK, Liu V, Diwan HA, et al. Atopic dermatitis. In: Dermatopathology: high-yield pathology. Philadelphia: Elsevier Saunders; 2011; with permission.)

Table 8
Prevention and treatment of atopic dermatitis

Prevention	Management of Symptoms
• Avoidance of triggers such as heat, dryness, stress, chemicals • Skin hydration with emollients, lotions	• Control itching using antihistamines • Control skin inflammation using topical corticosteroids, tacrolimus/pimecrolimus, ultraviolet B (UVB), psoralen, and ultraviolet A (PUVA) light therapy • Control infection with antibiotics against *Staphylococcus aureus*

Patient education by counseling patients on the medical, nutritional, and psychological issues surrounding their eczema has been proven to improve outcomes.

REFERENCES

1. Austen K. Chapter 317. Allergies, anaphylaxis, and systemic mastocytosis. In: Longo DL, Fauci AS, Kasper DL, et al, editors. Harrison's principles of internal medicine. New York: McGraw-Hill; 2012. p. 18e. Available at: http://accessmedicine. mhmedical.com/content.aspx?bookid=331&Sectionid=4072711.
2. Domino FJ, Baldor RA, Golding J, et al. Urticaria. In: Domino FJ, Baldor RA, Golding J, et al, editors. The 5-minute clinical consult. Philadelphia: Lippincott Williams & Wilkins; 2011. p. 1380–1.
3. Urticaria in DynaMed [database online]. EBSCO Information Services. 2015. Available at: http://web.a.ebscohost.com/dynamed/detail?vid=2&sid=a889 fde9-9658-42e7-96e5-445dd44f0ec9%40sessionmgr4005&hid=4207&bdata= JnNpdGU9ZHluYW1lZC1saXZlJnNjb3BlPXNpdGU%3d#db=dme&AN=T115276. Accessed March 15, 2015.
4. Bingham C. New Onset Urticaria. UpToDate; 2014. Web. St. Louis, MO, 1 Oct. 2014. Available at: http://www.uptodate.com/contents/new-onset-urticaria? source=search_result&search=new+onset+urticaria&selectedTitle=1%7E150# references.
5. Angioedema in DynaMed [database online]. EBSCO Information Services. 2015. Available at: http://web.a.ebscohost.com/dynamed/detail?vid=5&sid=a889fde9-9658-42e7-96e5-445dd44f0ec9%40sessionmgr4005&hid=4207&bdata=JnNpd GU9ZHluYW1lZC1saXZlJnNjb3BlPXNpdGU%3d#db=dme&AN=T566511. Accessed March 26, 2015.
6. Austen K. Chapter 317. Allergies, anaphylaxis, and systemic mastocytosis. In: Longo DL, Fauci AS, Kasper DL, et al, editors. Harrison's principles of internal medicine. 2012. p. 18e. Available at: http://accessmedicine.mhmedical.com. medjournal.hmc.psu.edu:2048/content.aspx?sectionid=79749806&bookid=1130& Resultclick=2&q=allergy anaphylaxis. Accessed March 15, 2015.
7. Atopic Dermatitis in Dynamed [database online]. EBSCO Information Services. 2015. Available at: http://web.b.ebscohost.com/dynamed/detail? vid=2&sid=e0154db2-7c89-4b74-9ef5-e17b1420267d%40sessionmgr112&hid= 118&bdata=JnNpdGU9ZHluYW1lZC1saXZlJnNjb3BlPXNpdGU%3d#db=dme& AN=T115212&anchor=sec-History-and-Physical. Accessed March 27, 2015.
8. Up to date Treatment of atopic dermatitis (eczema). 2015. Available at: http:// www.uptodate.com/contents/treatment-of-atopic-dermatitiseczema?source= search_result&search=atopic+dermatitis&selectedTitle=1%7E150. Accessed March 29, 2015.
9. Le T. First aid for family medicine boards. 2nd edition. New York: Mc Graw- Hill Medical; 2013.
10. Bingham C, Zuraw B. An overview of angioededma: clinical features diagnosis and management. In UpToDate. Available at: http://www.uptodate.com/ contents/an-overview-of-angioedema-clinical-featuresdiagnosismanagement? source=search_result&search=angioedema&selectedTitle=1%7E150#H25. Accessed March 25, 2015.

Bacterial Skin Infections

Fadi Ibrahim, MD[a],*, Tariq Khan, MD[a], George G.A. Pujalte, MD[b]

KEYWORDS

- Impetigo • Erysipelas • Cellulitis • Abscess
- Methicillin-resistant *Staphylococcus aureus*
- Methicillin-sensitive *Staphylococcus aureus*

KEY POINTS

- Impetigo involves the epidermis and is seen in children 2 to 5 years of age.
- Erysipelas involves the upper dermis and is most commonly caused by β-hemolytic streptococci.
- Cellulitis involves the deeper dermis and subcutaneous fat and is most commonly implicated by *Staphylococcus aureus* and GAS. It can be divided into nonpurulent and purulent cellulitis and treatment is based on extent of infection and risk factors.
- Abscesses involve the dermis and deeper skin tissues as a result of pus formation. Incision and drainage is the primary treatment.

INTRODUCTION

The integumentary system is an integral part of the immune system, serving as the first line of defense against bacterial infections.[1] The most common factor leading to the development of skin and soft tissue infection (SSTI) involves a breach of this barrier. A multitude of conditions can arise from this process differing mainly by the depth and extent of skin involvement. **Fig. 1** provides a graphical illustration of various SSTIs and their localization to various layers within the skin.

[a] Family Medicine, Mount Sinai Hospital, 1500 s California avenue, Chicago, IL 60608, USA;
[b] Family Medicine and Sports Medicine, Department of Family Medicine, Mayo Clinic, 4500 San Pablo Road, Jacksonville, FL 32224, USA
* Corresponding author.
E-mail address: fadi.ibrahim07@gmail.com

Prim Care Clin Office Pract 42 (2015) 485–499
http://dx.doi.org/10.1016/j.pop.2015.08.001
0095-4543/15/$ – see front matter © 2015 Elsevier Inc. All rights reserved.
primarycare.theclinics.com

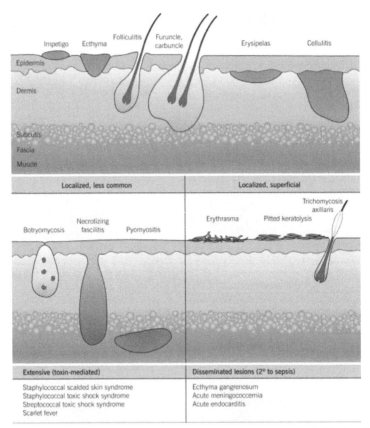

Fig. 1. Categorization of bacterial infections by depth and extent of skin involvement. More common, localized infections are depicted first; these infections are often secondary to *Staphylococcus aureus* or group A streptococci. (*From* Bolognia JL, Schaffer JV, Duncan KO, et al. Bacterial diseases. In: Dermatology essentials. Philadelphia: Elsevier; 2014. p. 574–90; with permission.)

IMPETIGO

Impetigo is a superficial soft tissue skin infection involving the epidermis. Nonbullous and bullous impetigo constitute the different types of impetigo. Pathogenesis includes primary (direct bacterial invasion of intact skin) or secondary "impetiginization" (bacterial infection of compromised skin flora). Common causes of alterations in the normal skin flora include abrasions, trauma, insect bites, eczema, and scabies. The most common organisms isolated include group A hemolytic streptococci and *Staphylococcus aureus*. Impetigo has increased occurrence in close contact, warm, and humid environments. Predisposing factors include lack of hygiene, poverty, and cramped areas.[2–5]

Evaluation and Work-Up

Nonbullous and bullous impetigo are differentiated easily based on several characteristic features. **Fig. 2** and **Table 1** summarize the key differences of these conditions.

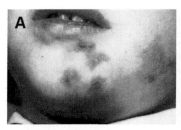 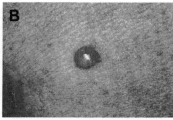

Fig. 2. (A) Impetigo. Note that the vesicles are covered by a golden crust. These perioral lesions are at a characteristic site. (B) Bullous impetigo. ([A] *Courtesy of* Dr R.A. Marsden, St. George's Hospital, London; and *From* Ferri FF. Bacterial skin infections. In: Ferri's color atlas and text of clinical medicine. 1st edition. Philadelphia: Saunders Elsevier; 2009. p. 134–42; with permission; and [B] *From* White G, Cox N. Diseases of the skin. 2nd edition. St Louis (MO): Mosby; 2006; with permission.)

Table 1 Summary of nonbullous impetigo versus bullous impetigo		
	Nonbullous Impetigo (Crusted)	**Bullous Impetigo**
Occurrence	Most common; 70% of all cases	Less common
Age	Any age	Most common in children ages 2–5 y
Organism	*Staphylococcus aureus* alone, or in combination with group A streptococcus, responsible for about 80% of cases	Most commonly caused by *S aureus*
Distribution	Most commonly affects the limbs and face	Occurs in such regions as the diaper area, axillae, and neck
Skin pattern	Yellowish crust that is, honey-colored	Erythematous, shiny wet base
Regional lymphadenopathy	Present	Absent
Treatment	Topical or oral therapy	Topical or oral therapy
Picture	See **Fig. 2**A	See **Fig. 2**B

Data from Refs.[2–4,6–8]

Management Strategies

All patients should be educated and adhere to good skin hygiene. Skin lesions should be kept clean and cleaned with soap and warm water. Removal of crusted lesions should be performed in nonbullous impetigo.

Pharmacologic Strategies

Topical antibiotics are the treatment of choice if lesions are local (<5 lesions). Systemic antibiotics are indicated for more widespread disease, when there are more than five lesions, fever, and/or regional lymphadenopathy. **Tables 2** and **3** summarize the key pharmacologic strategies used in treating these conditions.

Table 2 Topical antibiotics for impetigo		
Medication	**Adult Dose**	**Pediatric Dose**
Mupirocin	Apply to affected area three times daily for 3–5 d	

Data from Stevens DL, Bisno AL, Chambers HF, et al. Practice guidelines for the diagnosis and management of skin and soft tissue infections: 2014 update by the Infectious Diseases Society of America. Clin Infect Dis 2014;59:147.

Table 3 Oral Systemic antibiotics for impetigo		
Medication	**Adult Dose**	**Pediatric Dose**
Dicloxacillin	250–500 mg four times per day	25–50 mg/kg in four divided doses
Cephalexin	250–500 mg four times per day	25–50 mg/kg in three to four divided doses
If methicillin-resistant *Staphylococcus aureus* is suspected or confirmed		
Clindamycin	300–450 mg four times daily	20 mg/kg/d in three divided doses
Trimethoprim- sulfamethoxazole	1–2 double-strength tablets twice per day	8–12 mg/kg (trimethoprim) per day in two divided doses

Data from Stevens DL, Bisno AL, Chambers HF, et al. Practice guidelines for the diagnosis and management of skin and soft tissue infections: 2014 update by the Infectious Diseases Society of America. Clin Infect Dis 2014;59:147.

Follow-Up Care

Resolution of impetigo is expected after appropriate therapy. If no improvement is seen, failed therapy because of bacterial resistance or a different skin condition should be considered. Children are deemed fit to return to school 1 day after antibiotic therapy.

ERYSIPELAS

Erysipelas is a soft tissue infection involving the upper dermis. When compared with other soft tissue skin infections erysipelas has more distinct margins (**Fig. 3**, **Table 4**). β-Hemolytic streptococcus is the most common organism isolated.

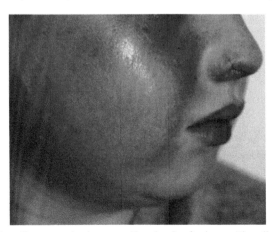

Fig. 3. Ill-defined erythema and edema on the cheek of a boy with cellulitis. (*Courtesy of* Brandon Newell, MD; from Lawrence HS, Nopper AJ. Superficial bacterial skin infections and cellulitis. In: Long SS, editor. Principles and practice of pediatric infectious diseases. 4th edition. Philadelphia: Churchill Livingstone; 2012. p. 427–35; with permission.)

Table 4 Summary of erysipelas characteristics	
	Erysipelas
Age	Any age
Organism	β-Hemolytic streptococci is most common organism
Distribution	Commonly affected areas include the face, ears, and lower extremities.
Skin pattern	Distinct margins of demarcation associated with warmth, erythema, and edema
Regional lymphadenopathy	Present
Treatment	Oral or parental therapy
Picture	See **Fig. 3**

Data from Stevens DL, Bisno AL, Chambers HF, et al. Practice guidelines for the diagnosis and management of skin and soft tissue infections: 2014 update by the Infectious Diseases Society of America. Clin Infect Dis 2014;59:147; and Bisno AL, Stevens DL. Streptococcal infections of skin and soft tissues. N Engl J Med 1996;334(4):240.

Predisposing risk factors include impaired venous or lymphatic drainage, and patients whom are immunocompromised.

Management Strategies

Elevation of the affected area should be performed if applicable, to promote venous/lymphatic drainage. Underlying predisposing conditions should be addressed. The skin should be sufficiently hydrated and dryness should be prevented. Compression stockings and diuretic therapy should be started to help improve the edema and promote lymphatic drainage.

Pharmacologic Strategies

Oral antibiotic is indicated; however, in severe cases of erysipelas, parenteral therapy may be warranted. **Table 5** summarizes the front-line antimicrobials used in treating erysipelas.

Table 5 Antimicrobial therapy for erysipelas		
	Adults	**Children Age >28 d**
Oral therapy		
Penicillin	500 mg orally every 6 h	25–50 mg/kg/d orally in three or four doses
Amoxicillin	500 mg orally every 8 h	25–50 mg/kg/d orally in three doses
Parenteral therapy		
Ceftriaxone	1 g intravenously every 24 h	50–75 mg/kg/d intravenously in one or two doses

Data from Stevens DL, Bisno AL, Chambers HF, et al. Practice guidelines for the diagnosis and management of skin and soft tissue infections: 2014 update by the Infectious Diseases Society of America. Clin Infect Dis 2014;59:147.

Follow-Up Care

Improvement is usually observed within 24 to 72 hours of antibiotic therapy. If no improvement is seen, failed therapy should be considered, and this is usually caused by bacterial resistance or a different skin condition.

CELLULITIS

Cellulitis represents a skin infection involving the deeper dermis and subcutaneous fat. The diagnosis is primarily clinical and depends on the appearance of the skin. As such, good physical examination techniques are paramount to establishing a diagnosis and identifying emergency conditions that require an immediate intervention.

Microbiology

The most common pathogens implicated in cellulitis include *S aureus* and group A streptococci (GAS). The best estimates place the rate of *S aureus* cellulitis at approximately 50% and GAS at approximately 27%.[9] The understanding of the prevalence of the microorganisms involved in causing cellulitis is limited because of the low yield of cultures from cellulitis. Less common causes of cellulitis are usually implicated in special clinical circumstances. **Table 6** summarize several unique circumstances and the pathogens implicated in these situations. Regardless of circumstances *S aureus* and GAS must be suspected in all patients with cellulitis.

Table 6
Cellulitis pathogens associated with particular epidemiology

Exposure	Pathogens
Dog bite	*Pasteurella multocida*, *Capnocytophaga* sp, mixed aerobic, and anaerobic flora
Cat bite	*P multocida*, mixed aerobic and anaerobic flora
Fish exposure	*Mycobacterium marinum*, *Erysipelothrix rhusiopathiae*, *Streptococcus iniae*
Salt water	*Vibrio vulnificus*
Fresh water	*Aeromonas hydrophilia*, *Edwardsiella tarda*, *Chromobacterium violaceum*, protothecosis
Cirrhosis	*V vulnificus* from raw seafood consumption; gram-negative rods
Intravenous drug use	*Eikenella corrodens* and other oral flora, *Pseudomonas aeruginosa* and other gram-negative rods, anaerobes including *Clostridium* sp
Neutropenia	*P aeruginosa* and other gram-negative rods fungi

Data from Stevens DL, Bisno AL, Chambers HF, et al. Practice guidelines for the diagnosis and management of skin and soft tissue infections: 2014 update by the Infectious Diseases Society of America. Clin Infect Dis 2014;59:147.

Methicillin-Resistant Staphylococcus aureus Versus Methicillin-Sensitive Staphylococcus aureus

The discovery of penicillin in 1928 and the subsequent widespread use of antibiotics heralded the era of antibiotic resistance. In 1961, the first case of *S aureus* resistant to conventional antibiotics was documented. This was deemed methicillin-resistant *S aureus* (MRSA). In the following decades, MRSA became more prevalent throughout the United States and Europe. Resistance giving rise to MRSA arose from the production of altered penicillin-binding proteins conferring lower pathogen affinities for β-lactam groups.

The 2011 Infectious Disease Society of America clinical practice guidelines for MRSA describe MRSA cellulitis as an infection involving purulence. Purulent cellulitis encompasses a process that began as an abscess resulting in secondary cellulitis or as a cellulitis with secondary purulence, purulent drainage, or exudate in the absence of a drainable abscess.[12]

Evaluation/Work-Up

Patient history

Patients generally present with localized erythema that is generally confluent (**Fig. 4**). Patients often complain of blanching with associated swelling, warmth, and tenderness of the involved area. Lymphangitis with tender regional lymphadenopathy is

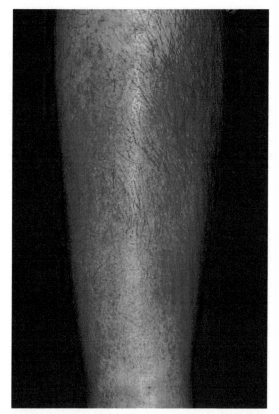

Fig. 4. Cellulitis. An early case with diffuse erythema and minimal swelling. Pain was elicited with palpation. (*From* Habif TP, Campbell JL, Chapman MS, et al. Bacterial infections. In: Skin disease. 3rd edition. Philadelphia: Saunders; 2011. p. 154–83; with permission.)

Box 1
Risk factors for cellulitis
Immunocompromised patients
Edema caused by venous insufficiency
Edema caused by lymphatic obstruction; this is particularly evident following surgery.
History of cellulitis: prior episode of cellulitis, especially of the lower extremity, increases likelihood of recurrent infections
Intravenous drug use
Edema caused by venous insufficiency
Data from Refs.[13–17]

common. Several factors can predispose an individual to developing cellulitis. Some of the factors commonly seen in clinical practice are listed in **Box 1**.

Physical examination

Initial examination should focus on determining the extent of disease. Patients' skin should be carefully examined for breaches, because they may often be small and unapparent. When a distal extremity is involved, the distal web spaces should be carefully examined for superficial bacterial or fungal infection, such as tinea pedis. The examiner should delineate the affected area with a marking pen to allow for evaluation of further progression after the initiation of therapy. It is important to note whether the infection is by nature purulent or nonpurulent, because this affects the course of treatment. On occasion, cellulitis may also cause deeper necrosis, resulting in dermal and subcutaneous abscess formation, fasciitis, and myonecrosis. The presence of certain physical examination findings should prompt a consideration of other diagnoses. Pain in the absence of erythema; pain out of proportion to the appearance of the local area; crepitus, a rare sign that signifies gas-forming pathogens; and macular erythema followed by diffuse epidermal exfoliation should raise concern for staphylococcal scaled skin syndrome. **Fig. 5** depicts epidermolytic toxins leading to separation of the epidermis beneath the granular cell layer.

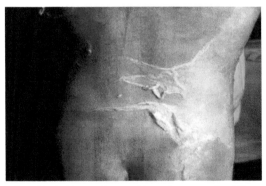

Fig. 5. Staphylococcal scalded skin syndrome. Note the extensive blistering. (*From* Ferri FF. Bacterial skin infections. In: Ferri's color atlas and text of clinical medicine. 1st edition. Philadelphia: Saunders Elsevier; 2009. p. 134–42; with permission.)

Imaging and additional testing

Routine laboratory tests, such as blood cultures, needle aspirations, or punch biopsies, are rare in the setting of mild infection. Various studies have shown the following: blood cultures are positive in less than 5% of cases,[18] culture results from needle aspiration vary from less than or equal to 5% to 40%,[18–25] and culture of punch biopsy specimens yields a pathogen in 20% to 30% of cases.[18–26]

White blood cell count with differential depicts leukocytosis with neutrophilia. If the antibiotic chosen is appropriate, the patient's fever and white blood cell count should respond. Imaging modalities in the setting of cellulitis are most commonly used to rule out abscess or diagnoses requiring emergent intervention described previously. The most common feature of cellulitis seen on MRI or ultrasound is subcutaneous tissue thickening.

Management Strategies

Management of cellulitis involves a multifaceted approach including a thorough evaluation and treatment of underlying conditions, supportive measures, and medications.

Treatment Strategies

The approach to antibiotic selection for treatment of cellulitis depends on whether the clinical presentation consists of purulent or nonpurulent cellulitis. According to the 2011 Infectious Disease Society of America clinical practice guidelines, purulent cellulitis is potentially attributable to *S aureus* and should be managed with empiric therapy for infection caused by MRSA, pending culture results. Empiric therapy for infection caused by β-hemolytic streptococci is likely not necessary.

Most patients develop mild cellulitis and can be treated with oral antibiotics. Inpatient admission for initial treatment with parenteral antibiotics should be considered for

- Patients with signs of systemic toxicity (hypotension) or erythema that has progressed rapidly
- Hypotension and/or the following laboratory findings
  - Elevated creatinine level
  - Elevated creatine phosphokinase level (two to three times the upper limit of normal)
  - C-reactive protein level greater than 13 mg/L (123.8 mmol/L)
  - Low serum bicarbonate level
  - Marked left shift on the complete blood count with differential

Pharmacologic Strategies: Nonpurulent

Pharmacologic stratreges for the treatment of nonpurulent cellulitis are detailed in **Table 7**. Empiric coverage for MRSA should be considered in patients with risk

Table 7
Empiric antimicrobial therapy for nonpurulent cellulitis (including β-hemolytic streptococci and methicillin-sensitive *Staphylococcus aureus*, but not MRSA)

	Adults	Children Age >28 d
Oral therapy		
Dicloxacillin	500 mg orally every 6 h	25–50 mg/kg/d orally in four doses
Cephalexin	500 mg orally every 6 h	25–50 mg/kg/d orally in three or four doses
Clindamycin	300–450 mg orally every 6–8 h	20–30 mg/kg/d orally in four doses
Intravenous therapy		
Cefazolin	1–2 g intravenously every 8 h	100 mg/kg/d intravenously in three or four doses
Oxacillin	2 g intravenously every 4 h	150–200 mg/kg/d intravenously in four or six doses
Nafcillin	2 g intravenously every 4 h	150–200 mg/kg/d intravenously in four or six doses
Clindamycin	600–900 mg intravenously every 8 h	25–40 mg/kg/d intravenously in three or four doses

Data from Refs.[5,10,11]

factors for MRSA infection and in communities where the prevalence of MRSA is greater than 30%. Pharmacological treatment strateges under these circumstances are discussed in **Table 8**. Refer to **Box 2** for a review of risk factors for MRSA infections.[5,27–31]

Box 2
Risk factors for MRSA colonization

Recent hospitalization

Residence in a long-term care facility

Recent antibiotic therapy

Hemodialysis

Military service

Prolonged hospital stay

Diabetes

Sharing sports equipment

Human immunodeficiency virus infection

Men who have sex with men

Injection drug use

Incarceration

Sharing needles, razors, or other sharp objects

Data from Refs.[5,10,27–29]

Table 8
Options for empiric oral therapy for treatment of both MRSA and GAS

Antibiotic	Adult Dose	Pediatric Dose (Children >28 d)
Clindamycin	300–450 mg orally three times daily	40 mg/kg/d orally divided in three or four doses
Amoxicillin and trimethoprim-sulfamethoxazole	500 mg orally three times daily	25–50 mg/kg/d orally divided in three doses
	1 double-strength tablet orally twice daily	8–12 mg trimethoprim component/kg/d orally divided in two doses
Amoxicillin and doxycycline	500 mg orally three times daily	25–50 mg/kg/d orally divided in three doses
	100 mg orally twice daily	≤45 kg: 4 mg/kg/d orally divided in two doses >45 kg: 100 mg orally twice daily
Amoxicillin and minocycline	500 mg orally three times daily	25–50 mg/kg/d orally divided in three doses
	200 mg once, then 100 mg orally twice daily	4 mg/kg orally once, then 4 mg/kg/d divided in two doses
Linezolid	600 mg orally twice daily	<12 y: 30 mg/kg/d orally divided in three doses ≥12 y: 600 mg orally twice daily
Tedizolid	200 mg orally once daily	—

Data from Refs.[5,10,27–29]

Pharamacolic Strateges: Purulent

Refer to **Tables 9** and **10** for a review of the treatment of purulent cellulitis and the appropriate antibiotic coverage.

Table 9 Oral antibiotics for infections caused by MRSA		
Antibiotic	**Adult Dose**	**Pediatric Dose (Children >28 d)**
Clindamycin	300–450 mg orally three times daily	40 mg/kg/d orally divided in three or four doses
Trimethoprim-sulfamethoxazole	1 double-strength tablet orally twice daily	8–12 mg trimethoprim component/kg/d orally divided in two doses
Doxycycline	100 mg orally twice daily	≤45 kg: 4 mg/kg/d orally divided in two doses >45 kg: 100 mg orally twice daily
Minocycline	200 mg orally once, then 100 mg orally twice daily	4 mg/kg orally once, then 4 mg/kg/d divided in two doses
Linezolid	600 mg orally twice daily	<12 y: 30 mg/kg/d orally divided in three doses ≥12 y: 600 mg orally twice daily
Tedizolid	200 orally once daily	—

Adapted from Liu C, Bayer A, Cosgrove SE, et al. Clinical practice guidelines by the Infectious Diseases Society of America for the treatment of methicillin-resistant *Staphylococcus aureus* infections in adults and children. Clin Infect Dis 2011;52:e18.

Table 10 Parenteral antibiotics for infections caused by MRSA	
Antibiotic	**Adult Dose**
Vancomycin	15–20 mg/kg/dose every 8–12 h, not to exceed 2 g per dose
Daptomycin	
Skin and soft tissue infection	4 mg/kg IV once daily
Bacteremia	6 mg/kg IV once daily
Linezolid	600 mg IV (or orally) twice daily
Ceftaroline	600 mg IV every 12 h
Dalbavancin (for skin and soft tissue infection)	1 g IV on Day 1, followed by 500 mg IV on Day 8
Tedizolid (for skin and soft tissue infection)	200 mg IV (or orally) twice daily
Telavancin	10 mg/kg once daily

Abbreviation: IV, intravenously.

Adapted from Stevens DL, Herr D, Lampiris H, et al. Linezolid versus vancomycin for the treatment of methicillin-resistant *Staphylococcus aureus* infections. Clin Infect Dis 2002;34:1481; and Choice of antibacterial drugs. Treat Guidel Med Lett 2007;5:33.

Nonpharmacologic Strategies

Cool, sterile saline dressings decrease the local pain and are particularly indicated in the presence of bullous lesions. The application of moist heat may aid in the localization of an abscess in association with cellulitis. Optimal management of predisposing conditions, when present, should be an integral part of the treatment plan.

Self-Management Strategies

Affected areas should be elevated, facilitating gravity-dependent drainage of edema and inflammatory mediators. Additionally, the skin should be sufficiently hydrated to avoid dryness and cracking.

Evaluation, Adjustment, Recurrence

Patients with cellulitis should receive interval evaluations and follow-up care to evaluate for improvement of disease. If symptoms fail to improve within 24 to 72 hours of initiating antibiotics, one should consider the possibility of failed therapy or a different skin condition.

ABSCESSES

Abscesses are collections of pus within the dermis and deeper skin tissues. They are often caused by a progression of skin infections. An abscess generally begins when bacteria multiply within a contained space, such as beneath the epidermis or the lumen of a hair follicle. Neutrophils are drawn to the site of infection, leading to the development of purulence through the actions of various cytokines and bacterial toxins. The overlying epidermis prevents drainage leading to the development of an abscess. Rarely, sterile abscesses can occur in the setting of injected irritants, such as in intravenous drug abuse.

Evaluation/Work-Up

Patient history

In essence, any process leading to a breach in the skin barrier can also predispose to the development of a skin abscess. Individuals in close contact with others who have active infection with skin abscesses, furuncles, and carbuncles are at an increased risk. Individuals exposed to whirlpool footbaths at nail salons are at risk for mycobacterial furunculosis. Given that abscesses are most often caused by progression of cellulitis, please refer to **Box 1** for a review of the risk factors implicated in their development.

Physical examination

Skin abscesses manifest as painful, tender, fluctuant, and erythematous nodules, frequently surmounted by a pustule and surrounded by a rim of erythematous swelling (**Fig. 6**). Spontaneous drainage of purulent material may occur, and regional adenopathy may be observed.

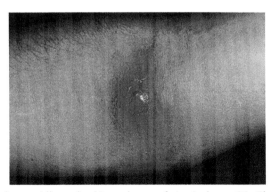

Fig. 6. A furuncle has rapidly evolved in a plaque of atopic dermatitis. The center is swollen and soft and will soon rupture and exude purulent material. (*From* Habif TP, Campbell JL, Chapman MS, et al. Bacterial infections. In: Skin disease. 3rd edition. Philadelphia: Saunders; 2011. p. 154–83; with permission.)

Imaging and additional testing

Bedside ultrasound examination is the best option for the differentiation of abscess from cellulitis in challenging situations. Abscesses are seen as hypoechoic areas with posterior acoustic enhancement. The hypoechoic areas usually represent pus and may be heterogeneous with some bright signals. Before the emergence of MRSA, microbiologic cultures were not obtained routinely. In the era of antibiotic resistance, cultures are useful in guiding therapy and prevention.

Management Strategies

Incision and drainage is the primary and definitive treatment of abscesses. Antibiotic coverage is appropriate when there is underlying cellulitis.

Pharmacologic Strategies

According to Infectious Disease Society of America guidelines, antibiotic therapy is recommended for abscesses associated with the conditions shown in **Box 3**.

Box 3
Conditions in which antibiotic therapy is recommended for abscesses

Severe or extensive disease (eg, involving multiple sites of infection)

Rapid progression in presence of associated cellulitis

Signs and symptoms of systemic illness

Associated comorbidities or immunosuppression

Extremes of age

Abscess in an area difficult to drain (eg, face, hand, and genitalia)

Associated septic phlebitis

Lack of response to incision and drainage alone (A-III)

Data from Stevens DL, Bisno AL, Chambers HF, et al. Practice guidelines for the diagnosis and management of skin and soft tissue infections: 2014 update by the Infectious Diseases Society of America. Clin Infect Dis 2014;59:147.

Nonpharmacologic Strategies

Cool, sterile saline dressings decrease the local pain and are particularly indicated in the presence of bullous lesions. The application of moist heat may aid in the localization of an abscess in association with cellulitis. Optimal management of predisposing conditions, when present, should be an integral part of the treatment plan.

Self-Management Strategies

Self-management strategies for abscesses are limited to maintaining cleanliness and the application of warm compresses.

Evaluation, Adjustment, Recurrence

Recurrent infection may occur as a result of epidemiologic risk factors, such as host immunosuppression. Efforts should be made in these circumstances to treat the underlying cause. Patients with acquired immunosuppressive should be optimized on appropriate therapies to prevent recurring infections. Skin abscesses are rarely fatal, and most eventually rupture through the epidermis and drain spontaneously.

SUMMARY

SSTIs are a common condition seen in inpatient and outpatient settings. Primary care providers should be able to diagnose, manage, and provide appropriate follow-up care for these frequently seen skin infections. Each infection is characterized based on the extent of skin involvement. More superficial involvement is seen in impetigo and erysipelas involving the outer epidermis and upper dermis, respectively. Deeper layer involvement is seen in cellulitis and abscesses. Many of these conditions share similar management strategies, including prompt initiation of antibiotics and incision and drainage when indicated. Wound care and follow-up care are critical parts in the management of SSTIs to ensure appropriate resolution and in the prevention of further disease progression.

REFERENCES

1. Agency for Healthcare Research and Quality (AHRQ). Medical expenditure panel survey. Available at: http://www.meps.ahrq.gov/mepsweb/. Accessed June 3, 2015.
2. Hartman-Adams H, Banvard C, Juckett G. Impetigo: diagnosis and treatment. Am Fam Physician 2014;90(4):229–35.
3. Dajani AS, Ferrieri P, Wannamaker LW. Natural history of impetigo. II. Etiologic agents and bacterial interactions. J Clin Invest 1972;51:2863.
4. Hirschmann JV. Impetigo: etiology and therapy. Curr Clin Top Infect Dis 2002;22: 42–51.
5. Stevens DL, Bisno AL, Chambers HF, et al. Practice guidelines for the diagnosis and management of skin and soft tissue infections: 2014 update by the Infectious Diseases Society of America. Clin Infect Dis 2014;59:147.
6. Rhody C. Bacterial infections of the skin. Prim Care 2000;27:459–73.
7. Schachner L, Gonzalez A. Diagnosis and treatment of impetigo. J Am Acad Dermatol 1989;20:132.
8. Dagan R. Impetigo in childhood: changing epidemiology and new treatments. Pediatr Ann 1993;22:235–40.
9. Chira S, Miller LG. *Staphylococcus aureus* is the most common identified cause of cellulitis: a systematic review. Epidemiol Infect 2010;138(3):313–7.
10. Swartz MN. Clinical practice. Cellulitis. N Engl J Med 2004;350:904.
11. Pallin DJ, Binder WD, Allen MB, et al. Clinical trial: comparative effectiveness of cephalexin plus trimethoprim-sulfamethoxazole versus cephalexin alone for treatment of uncomplicated cellulitis: a randomized controlled trial. Clin Infect Dis 2013;56:1754.
12. Liu C, Bayer A, Cosgrove SE, et al. Clinical practice guidelines by the Infectious Diseases Society of America for the treatment of methicillin-resistant staphylococcus aureus infections in adults and children. Clin Infect Dis 2011;52(3):e18–35.
13. Dupuy A, Benchikhi H, Roujeau JC, et al. Risk factors for erysipelas of the leg (cellulitis): case-control study. BMJ 1999;318(7198):1591.
14. McNamara DR, Tleyjeh IM, Berbari EF, et al. A predictive model of recurrent lower extremity cellulitis in a population-based cohort. Arch Intern Med 2007;167(7):709.
15. Dan M, Heller K, Shapira I, et al. Incidence of erysipelas following venectomy for coronary artery bypass surgery. Infection 1987;15(2):107.
16. Baddour LM, Bisno AL. Recurrent cellulitis after saphenous venectomy for coronary bypass surgery. Ann Intern Med 1982;97(4):493.
17. Simon MS, Cody RL. Cellulitis after axillary lymph node dissection for carcinoma of the breast. Am J Med 1992;93(5):543.

18. Perl B, Gottehrer NP, Raveh D, et al. Cost-effectiveness of blood cultures for adult patients with cellulitis. Clin Infect Dis 1999;29(6):1483.
19. Kielhofner MA, Brown B, Dall L. Influence of underlying disease process on the utility of cellulitis needle aspirates. Arch Intern Med 1988;148:2451.
20. Hook EW III, Hooton TM, Horton CA, et al. Microbiologic evaluation of cutaneous cellulitis in adults. Arch Intern Med 1986;146:295.
21. Sachs MK. The optimum use of needle aspiration in the bacteriologic diagnosis of cellulitis in adults. Arch Intern Med 1990;150:1907.
22. Leppard BJ, Seal DV, Colman G, et al. The value of bacteriology and serology in the diagnosis of cellulitis and erysipelas. Br J Dermatol 1985;112:559.
23. Sigurdsson AF, Gudmundsson S. The etiology of bacterial cellulitis as determined by fine-needle aspiration. Scand J Infect Dis 1989;21:537.
24. Newell PM, Norden CW. Value of needle aspiration in bacteriologic diagnosis of cellulitis in adults. J Clin Microbiol 1988;26:401.
25. Lebre C, Girard-Pipau F, Roujeau JC, et al. Value of fine-needle aspiration in infectious cellulitis. Arch Dermatol 1996;132:842.
26. Duvanel T, Auckenthaler R, Rohner P, et al. Quantitative cultures of biopsy specimens from cutaneous cellulitis. Arch Intern Med 1989;149:293.
27. Bernard P, Plantin P, Roger H, et al. Roxithromycin versus penicillin in the treatment of erysipelas in adults: a comparative study. Br J Dermatol 1992;127:155.
28. Martin JM, Green M, Barbadora KA, et al. Erythromycin-resistant group A streptococci in schoolchildren in Pittsburgh. N Engl J Med 2002;346:1200.
29. Treatment of community-associated MRSA infections. Med Lett Drugs Ther 2006;48:13.
30. Miller LG, Daum RS, Creech CB, et al. Clindamycin versus trimethoprim-sulfamethoxazole for uncomplicated skin infections. N Engl J Med 2015;372:1093.
31. Hepburn MJ, Dooley DP, Skidmore PJ, et al. Comparison of short-course (5 days) and standard (10 days) treatment for uncomplicated cellulitis. Arch Intern Med 2004;164:1669.

Superficial Fungal Infections

Neha Kaushik, MD[a],*, George G.A. Pujalte, MD[b], Stephanie T. Reese, DO[c]

KEYWORDS

- Superficial fungal infection • Tinea pedis • Tinea capitis • Tinea corporis
- Tinea barbae • Tinea versicolor • Candidiasis • Antifungal treatment

KEY POINTS

- Superficial fungal infections are caused by numerous fungi, which invade the skin, mucosal sites, and systemic body.
- Superficial fungal infections are caused by dermatophytes affecting keratinized epithelium, *Candida* sp, which infects warm areas, and *Malassezia* sp, which requires a warm and lipophilic environment in which to thrive.
- The fungal infections can have various presentations on the human body.
- Many treatment options are available, such as creams and oral antifungal agents.

INTRODUCTION

Superficial fungal infections are caused by many fungi, which can invade various aspects of the human body.[1-3] These infections include dermatophytes, which infect keratinized epithelium, hair follicles, and nail apparatus; *Candida* sp, which needs a warm, humid environment; *Malassezia* sp, which requires a humid microenvironment and lipids to grow; and *Trichosporon* sp and *Hortae* sp. Dermatophytes infect nonviable, keratinized cutaneous structures such as stratum corneum, nails, and hair.[1-3] An epidermal dermatophytosis infection is called *epidermomycosis*, dermatophytosis of hair and hair follicles is called *trichomycosis*, and dermatophytosis of the nail apparatus is called *onchomycosis*. Three genera of dermatophytes exist: *Trichophyton*

Disclosure Statement: The authors have nothing to disclose.
[a] PGY-3 Family Medicine Resident, Community Medicine Residency Program, Department of Family Medicine, Penn State Milton S. Hershey Medical Center, 500 University Drive, H154, PO Box 850, Hershey, PA 17033-0850, USA; [b] Family Medicine and Sports Medicine, Department of Family Medicine, Mayo Clinic, 4500 San Pablo Road, Jacksonville, FL 32224, USA; [c] Division of Primary Care, Family Medicine, Mayo Clinic Health System, 1921 Alice Street, Waycross, GA 31501, USA
* Corresponding author.
E-mail address: nkaushik@hmc.psu.edu

sp, *Microsporum* sp, and *Epidermophyton* sp. *Trichophyton rubrum* is the most common cause of epidermal dermatophytosis and onchomycosis.[4]

Transmission

Dermatophyte infections can be transmitted from person to person through fomites, transmitted from animals to humans, and, least commonly, acquired from soil. Predisposing factors for complicated dermatophyte infections include atopic diathesis, such as cell-mediated immune deficiency for *T rubrum*, prolonged immunosuppression with use of topical glucocorticoids, and systemic immunocompromised states.[4]

Classification

Dermatophytes are classified in several ways. There are many species of *Microsporum* and *Trichophyton* and one species of *Epidermophyton*. Dermatophytoses of keratinized epidermis include tinea facialis, tinea corporis, tinea cruris, tinea mannus, and tinea pedis. Dermatophytoses of nail apparatus include tinea unguium (toenails, fingernails). Dermatophytoses of hair and hair follicles (trichomycosis) include dermatophytic folliculitis, tinea capitis, and tinea barbae.

Diagnosis

It is important to recognize characteristic patterns of inflammation to diagnose fungal infections. The highest numbers of hyphae are located in the active border of infection, the best area to obtain a sample for potassium hydroxide examination. The active border is scaly, red, and slightly elevated. One can find vesicles in the active border when inflammation is intense. Many ways of obtaining a diagnosis exist through laboratory examinations.[5,6]

The most important test for the diagnosis of dermatophyte infection is direct visualization under microscopy of the branching hyphae in keratinized material. One should collect scale with a scalpel blade, place on the center of a microscopy slide, and cover with a coverslip. Potassium hydroxide, 5% to 20% solution, is applied at the edge of the coverslip. The preparation should be gently heated under low flame until bubbles begin to expand, clarifying the preparation. Potassium hydroxide dissolves the material that binds cells together but does not distort the epithelial cells or fungi. Under microscopy, dermatophytes will be recognized as septated, tubelike structures called *hyphae* and *mycelia*. A slight back-and-forth rotation of the focusing knob can aid in visualization of the entire segment of the hyphae, which may be at different depths.[5,6]

A Wood's lamp can be used to visualize hairs infected with *Microsporum* species, which fluoresce in a greenish color in a dark room. Fungal cultures are grown on Sabouraud's glucose medium, but it is usually not necessary to know the species of dermatophyte infecting the skin, as the same oral and topical agents are effective against all of them.

Distal and lateral subungual onchomycosis are best visualized using periodic acid-Schiff or methenamine silver stains, which are more sensitive than potassium hydroxide preparation or fungal culture.

TINEA PEDIS

Dermatophyte infections are classified by body regions. *Tinea* means fungus infection. As noted in **Fig. 1**, tinea pedis is the dermatophyte infection of the foot (athlete's foot). Warmth and sweating promote fungal growth. Tinea should be considered in the differential diagnosis of children with foot dermatitis.[7]

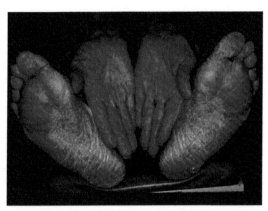

Fig. 1. Tinea pedis. (*From* Elewski BE, Hughey LC, Sobera JO, et al. Fungal diseases. In: Bolognia JL, Jorizzo JL, Schaffer JV, editors. Dermatology. 3rd edition. Philadelphia: Saunders; 2012; with permission.)

Locker room floors are a perfect environment for fungal growth. The use of communal baths creates an ideal condition for repeated exposure. The most common age range affected is late childhood to young adulthood, and males are more affected than females.

Tinea pedis can present with the classic ringworm pattern but most infections are found in toe webs or on the soles. The web between the fourth and fifth digits is commonly involved. The web can become dry, scaly, and fissured or white, macerated, and soggy. Itching is the most severe complaint with the removal of shoes and socks.[8] Overgrowth of the resident bacterial population is what determines the severity of this interdigital toe web infection, as the macerated part of the infection occurs as a result of the interaction between bacteria and fungus.

Dermatophytes initiate damage to stratum corneum and, by production of antibiotics, influence selection of a more antibiotic-resistant bacterial population, such as methicillin-resistant *Staphylococcus aureus* and group B *Streptococcus.* Diagnosis is obtained clinically. However, demonstration of hyphae on direct microscopy and isolation of dermatophytes on culture are also available.

Two feet-one hand syndrome involves dermatophyte infection of both feet, with tinea of one of the palms. Nail infection of the hands and feet can also be present. Most cases occur in men and *T rubrum* is the causative organism in most cases.[9]

The newest class of antifungal agents produces higher cure rates and rapid responses in dermatophyte infections. Topical antifungal preparations should be applied twice daily in the involved area optimally for 4 weeks, including 1 week after lesions are cleared. The topical agents are in the class of imidazoles and include clotrimazole, miconazole, and ketoconazole. One can also use terbinafine, 1% cream. If the infection becomes extensive or fails to respond to topical preparations, systemic antifungal agents should be used, such as terbinafine, 250 mg tablet daily for 2 weeks; itraconazole, 200 mg twice daily for 1 week; or fluconazole, 150 mg once weekly for 2-6 weeks.[10–13]

Recurrence is prevented by wearing wider shoes and expanding the web space with a small strand of lamb's wool. Powders will absorb moisture and should be applied to the feet rather than to the shoes.

Pitted Keratolysis

Pitted keratolysis is a disease that mimics tinea pedis and is an eruption of the weight-bearing surfaces of the soles. Common sites of onset include pressure-bearing areas such as ventral aspect of the toe, the ball of the foot, and the heel. Hyperhidrosis is the most common observed symptom. Malodor and sliminess of the skin are also key features. This disease is bacterial in origin but is often misinterpreted as fungal. Common characteristics include many circular or longitudinal, punched-out depressions in the skin surface. Hyperhidrosis, moist socks, and immersion of feet favor its development. Treatment includes promotion of dryness and frequent changing of socks. Rapid clearing occurs with application of 20% aluminum chloride twice a day. Other options include alcohol-based benzoyl peroxide, acne medications such as topical erythromycin solution and clindamycin solution, and mupirocin ointment.[14,15]

TINEA CRURIS

Tinea of the groin, or jock itch, medically referred to as *tinea cruris*, occurs in warm weather such as summertime after excessive sweating and wearing wet clothing. The promoting factor is the presence of a warm, moist environment. Men generally are affected more than women, and children will rarely get tinea of the groin. Itching becomes worse as moisture gathers and macerates the intertriginous area.

Lesions are usually unilateral and start in the crural fold. A half-moon–shaped plaque forms as well-defined scaling, and, occasionally, a vesicular border advances out of the crural fold onto the thigh. The skin within the border will turn red-brown, is less scaly, and can develop red papules. The infection can travel to the buttocks and gluteal cleft area. For proper diagnosis, specimens for potassium hydroxide examination should be taken from the advancing scaling border.[16]

Differential diagnoses for tinea cruris include intertrigo and erythrasma. Intertrigo is a red, macerated, half-moon–shaped plaque that resembles tinea of the groin and extends to an equal extent onto the groin and down the thigh, forming after moisture accumulates in the crural fold. Obesity and moisture are contributing factors to this inflammatory process, which can be infected with a mixed flora of bacteria, fungi, and yeast. Painful longitudinal fissures occur in the crease of the crural fold. Groin intertrigo recurs after treatment unless weight and moisture can be well controlled.

Erythrasma is a bacterial infection caused by *Corynebacterium minutissimum*, which can be confused with tinea cruris because of the similar, half-moon–shaped plaque. It is different in that it is noninflammatory, is uniformly brown and scaly, and has no advancing border. This organism produces porphyrins, which fluoresce coral-red with Wood's light, whereas tinea cruris does not fluoresce. Common sites of erythrasma are in the fourth interdigital toe space along with in the inframammary fold of the axillae. Erythrasma is treated with erythromycin, 250 mg 4 times a day for 5 days, or clarithromycin, single 1-g dose, or topically with miconazole, clotrimazole, or econazole creams.[17]

Tinea cruris lesions can respond quickly to antifungal creams, but they should be applied twice daily for 10 days at a minimum. Moist intertriginous areas can be mixed with dermatophytes, other fungi, or bacteria, and completion of full treatment duration is vital.

Residual inflammation from intertrigo can be treated with group V through VII topical steroids twice a day for 5 to 10 days. Betamethasone dipropionate/clotrimazole solutions or creams can be used for initial treatment if lesions are red, inflamed, and itchy. Systemic therapy is occasionally needed. Tinea cruris is appropriately treated with 50 to 100 mg fluconazole daily or 150 mg once weekly for 2 to 3 weeks, by 100 mg itraconazole daily for 2 weeks or 200 mg daily for 7 days, or by 250 mg terbinafine daily for 1 to 2 weeks. Griseofulvin 250 mg three times daily for 14 days is also effective.[18,19] Summary of treatment is shown in **Table 1**.

TINEA CORPORIS

Tinea of the face, (excluding the beard area in men), trunk, and limbs is called tinea corporis or ringworm of the body (**Fig. 2**). This disease occurs at any age and is more common in warm climates. A broad range of manifestations exist with lesions varying in size, degree of inflammation, and depth of involvement. This variability occurs because of the differences in host immunity and the species of fungus.[16]

In the classic ringworm, lesions start off as flat, scaly spots that then develop a raised border that extends out at varying rates in all directions. The advancing, scaly border may have red, raised papules or vesicles while the central area becomes brown or hypopigmented and less scaly as the active border progresses outward. There may be just one ring that grows to a few centimeters in diameter and will self-resolve or several annular lesions that enlarge to cover large areas of the body surface. The larger lesions may be asymptomatic or mildly itchy. They can reach a certain size and persist for years without resolution. Clear, central areas of the larger lesions are yellow-brown and usually contain several red papules, whereas the borders are annular and very irregular.[16] Tinea corporis has become common in competitive wrestling. Most of the reported cases are caused by *Trichophyton tonsurans*, and person-to-person contact is the main culprit of transmission.[20]

Deep Inflammatory Lesions

Zoophilic fungi such as *Trichophyton verrucosum* from cattle may produce a very inflammatory skin infection. This infection is more common in northern regions where cattle are confined in close quarters in the winter season. The round, intensely inflamed lesion has a uniformly elevated, red, boggy, pustular surface. The pustules are follicular and represent deep penetration of the fungus into the hair follicle.

A fungal culture helps identify the animal source of the infection. A distinctive form of inflammatory tinea called *Majocchi's granuloma* is caused by *T rubrum* and was originally described as occurring on the lower leg of women who shave, but it is also seen

Table 1 Treatment for tinea cruris and erythrasma		
Disease	**Definition**	**Treatment**
Erythrasma	Bacterial infection	Erythromycin 250 mg qid × 5 d or Clarithromycin 1 g × 1 or Topical miconazole, clotrimazole, or econazole creams
Tinea cruris	Fungal infection at groin	Fluconazole 50–100 mg daily or Fluconazole 150 mg once weekly × 2–3 wk Itraconazole 100 mg daily × 2 wk Itraconazole 200 mg × 7 d Terbinafine 250 mg daily × 1–2 wk Griseofulvin 250 mg tid for 14 days

Adapted from Habif TB. Clinical dermatology: a color guide to diagnosis and therapy. Philadelphia: Mosby/Elsevier; 2004.

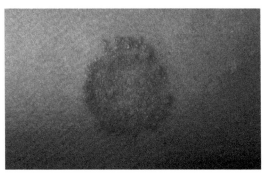

Fig. 2. Tinea corporis. (*From* Elewski BE, Hughey LC, Sobera JO, et al. Fungal diseases. In: Bolognia JL, Jorizzo JL, Schaffer JV, editors. Dermatology. 3rd edition. Philadelphia: Saunders; 2012; with permission.)

at other sites on men and children. The primary lesion is a follicular papulopustule or inflammatory nodule. Intracutaneous and subcutaneous granulomatous nodules arise from these initial inflammatory tinea infections. Lesions have necrotic areas containing fungal elements which are surrounded by epitheliod cells, giant cells, lymphocytes, and polymorphonuclear leukocytes, and are believed to be a result from rupturing of infected follicles into the dermis and subcutis.

The superficial lesions of tinea corporis respond to antifungal creams and typically require 2 weeks of twice-a-day treatment before a response is seen.[21–23] Treatment should continue 1 week after resolution of the infection. Those infections that are extensive or have red papules respond better to oral therapy.

Tinea corporis is treated by 150 mg to 200 mg of fluconazole once weekly for 2 to 4 weeks, by 200 mg itraconazole daily for 7 days, and by 250 mg terbinafine daily for 1 week.[21–23] Summary of treatment is shown in **Table 2**. Recurrence can be high with those having extensive superficial infections. Deep inflammatory lesions require 1 to 3 or more months of oral therapy.[21–23]

Inflammation can be reduced with wet Burrow's solution compresses, and bacterial infection is treated with appropriate oral antibiotics.

TINEA OF THE HAND

Tinea of the dorsal aspect of the hand, or tinea manuum, has all the features of tinea corporis. Tinea of the palm has the same appearance as the dry, diffuse, keratotic form of tinea on the soles. The dry keratotic form can be asymptomatic; hence,

Table 2 Treatment for tinea corporis	
Disease	**Treatment**
Tinea corporis	Fluconazole 150 – 200 mg once weekly for 2–4 weeks Intraconazole 200 mg × 7 days Terbinafine 250 mg daily for 1 week

Adapted from Habif TB. Clinical dermatology: a color guide to diagnosis and therapy. Philadelphia: Mosby/Elsevier; 2004.

patients may be unaware of the infection, attributing the dry, thick, scaly surface to hard physical labor. Tinea of the palms is frequently seen in association with tinea pedis. The usual pattern of infection involves 1 foot and 2 hands or 2 feet and 1 hand. Treatment is the same as for tinea pedis.

Tinea Incognito

Fungal infections that are treated with topical steroids often lose some of their characteristic features. Topical steroids decrease inflammation and give the false impression that the rash is improving while the fungus continues to thrive secondary to cortisone-induced immunologic changes. When treatment is stopped, the rash returns but in a different manner. Scaling at the margins can be absent. Diffuse erythema, diffuse scale, scattered pustules or papules, and brown hyperpigmentation may all result. A once localized process may have expanded greatly and the intensity of itching is variable.

Tinea incognito is most often seen on the groin, the face, and the dorsal aspect of the hand. Tinea infections of the hand are frequently misdiagnosed as eczema and treated with topical steroids. Hyphae are easily seen when scaling reappears.

TINEA OF THE SCALP

Tinea of the scalp, or tinea capitis, occurs most frequently in prepubertal children between 3 and 7 years of age and has several different presentations.[24] Anthropophilic species found in humans is the most likely species of dermatophyte to cause this infection. Tinea capitis, which can be visualized in **Fig. 3**, is most common in areas of poverty and crowded living conditions. The infection originates from contact with a pet or an infected person. Spores are shed in the air in the vicinity of the patient; hence, direct contact is not necessary for transmission. Tinea of the scalp is contagious by direct contact or from contaminated clothing.

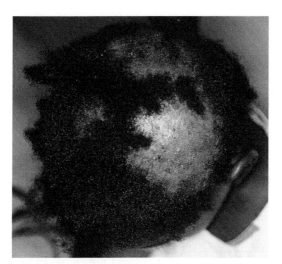

Fig. 3. Tinea capitis. (*From* Elewski BE, Hughey LC, Sobera JO, et al. Fungal diseases. In: Bolognia JL, Jorizzo JL, Schaffer JV, editors. Dermatology. 3rd edition. Philadelphia: Saunders; 2012; with permission.)

Large family size, crowding, and low socioeconomic status have a higher correlation with rates of fungal infections. Infectious particles shed from infected person can be viable for months. Common modes of transmission include infected persons, fallen hairs, animals, fomites (clothing, bedding, hairbrushes, combs, hats), and furniture. Untreated asymptomatic scalp infections in school children and adults are important contributing factors to disease transmission and reinfection. The asymptomatic carriage persists for an indefinite period.[25]

Three patterns of hair invasion exist: small-spored ectothrix, large-spored ectothrix, and large-spored endothrix. A summary of the patterns is shown in **Table 3**. The inflammatory response to infection is variable. A severe, inflammatory reaction with a boggy, indurated, tumorlike mass that exudes pus is called a *kerion*, and it represents a hypersensitivity reaction to fungus and heals with scarring and mild hair loss. One can also see cervical or occipital lymphadenopathy; the diagnosis of tinea capitis should be questioned if lymphadenopathy is not present.

Seborrheic dermatitis and psoriasis can often be confused with tinea of the scalp. Tinea amiantacea, a form of seborrheic dermatitis that occurs in children, is frequently misdiagnosed as tinea. Tinea amiantacea is a localized 2- to 8-cm patch of large, brown, polygonal-shaped scales that adheres to the scalp and mats the hair. The matted scale grows out, attached to the hair without much inflammation.

Summary of treatment is shown in **Table 4**. Griseofulvin is the current drug of choice in children. It is approved by the US Food and Drug Administration for treatment in children, has fewer known drug interactions, and is well tolerated. Dosages of 20 to 25 mg/kg/d are prescribed for 6 to 8 weeks. Safety, efficacy, and cost data favor terbinafine for treatment of *T tonsurans* infections. Shampoos containing 1% to 2.5% selenium sulfide, 1% to 2% zinc pyrithione, povidone-iodine, or ketoconazole 2% inhibit the growth of fungi. These agents are lathered and massaged adequately, then left on scalp for 5 minutes. They should be used 2 to 3 times each week during the course of treatment or longer.[26]

Trichophyton tonsurans

T tonsurans (large-spored endothrix) has been responsible for more than 90% of scalp ringworm in the United States. The occurrence rate is equal in boys and girls and most cases are seen in crowded inner cities in blacks or Hispanics. *T tonsurans* does not fluoresce and infects people of all ages. It remains viable for long periods of time on inanimate objects such as combs, brushes, blankets, and telephones. The peak incidence of infection occurs between 3 and 9 years of age.[27] This fungal infection does not resolve spontaneously and can result in a large population of infected carriers.[27]

Table 3 Patterns of hair invasion	
Patterns	**Description**
Small-spored ectothrix	Small pores randomly arranged in masses inside and on surface of hair shaft
Large-spored ectothrix	Chains of large spores inside and on surface on hair shaft
Large-spored endothrix	Chains of large spores, densely packed, within the hair

Adapted from Habif TB. Clinical dermatology: a color guide to diagnosis and therapy. Philadelphia: Mosby/Elsevier; 2004.

Table 4
Tinea capitis—oral drugs for treatment in children

Drug	Dosage	Duration
Griseofulvin (250-, 333-, and 500-mg tablets or suspension)	20–25 mg/kg/d (microsize formulation)	6–12 wk
	10–15 mg/kg/d (ultramicrosize formulation)	6–12 wk
Terbinafine (250-mg tablet)	Weight, 10–20 kg: 62.5 mg daily	4–6 wk
	Weight, 20–40 kg: 125 mg	4–6 wk
	Weight >40 kg: 250 mg	4–6 wk
Itraconazole (100-mg tablet or oral suspension)	3–5 mg/kg/d	4–6 wk
	5 mg/kg/d for 1 wk every month	2–3 mo
	3 mg/kg/d (oral suspension)	2–3 mo

Adapted from Habif TB. Clinical dermatology: a color guide to diagnosis and therapy. Philadelphia: Mosby/Elsevier; 2004.

TINEA OF THE BEARD

Fungal infection of the beard area, or tinea barbae should be thought of when inflammation is found in this region (**Fig. 4**). Bacterial folliculitis and inflammation secondary to ingrown hairs are common.

A positive culture for *Staphylococcus* sp does not rule out tinea, as purulent lesions can be infected secondarily with bacteria. A superficial infection pattern resembles the annular lesions of tinea corporis, whereas the deep follicular infection resembles bacterial folliculitis but is slower to evolve and usually restricted to one area of the beard. Tinea begins with a small group of follicular pustules, which, over time, becomes

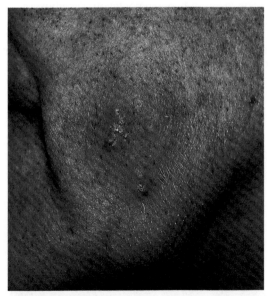

Fig. 4. Tinea barbae. (*From* Elewski BE, Hughey LC, Sobera JO, et al. Fungal diseases. In: Bolognia JL, Jorizzo JL, Schaffer JV, editors. Dermatology. 3rd edition. Philadelphia: Saunders; 2012; with permission.)

confluent with development of boggy, erythematous, tumorlike abscess covered with dense, superficial crust similar to fungal kerions seen in tinea capitis. Hairs can be removed at any stage of the infection and examined for hyphae. Zoophilic *Trichophyton mentagrophytes* and *T verrucosum* are the most common pathogens.

T verrucosum infection frequently is seen in farmers, as *T verrucosum* is transmitted from hides of dairy cattle and causes severe pustular eruptions on the face and neck. Treatment is the same as that of tinea capitis and requires oral agents, because creams do not penetrate depths of the hair follicle.

TINEA VERSICOLOR

Tinea versicolor (**Fig. 5**) is a common fungal infection of the skin caused by dimorphic lipophilic yeasts, *Pityrosporum orbiculare* and *Pityrosporum ovale*. Both organisms were previously known *as Malassezia furfur*.[28]

The organism is part of normal skin flora and appears in highest numbers where sebaceous activity is high. It lives within the stratum corneum and hair follicles where it feeds off free fatty acids and triglycerides.

Adrenalectomy, Cushing's disease, pregnancy, malnutrition, burns, corticosteroid therapy, immunosuppression, depressed cellular immunity, and oral contraceptives are a few predisposing factors that cause yeast to convert from the budding yeast form to its mycelial form, which leads to the formation of tinea versicolor. Disease can occur at any age but is more common during adolescence and young adulthood.[29,30]

Lesions begin as multiple small, circular macules of various colors (white, pink, or brown) that enlarge rapidly. Tinea versicolor infections produce a spectrum of clinical presentations including (1) red to fawn-colored macules, patches, or follicular papules that are caused by a hyperemic inflammatory response; (2) hypopigmented lesions; and (3) tan to dark brown macules and patches.

Melanocyte damage leads to hypopigmentation. Dicarboxylic acids produced by *Pityrosporum* sp can have a cytotoxic effect of melanocytes and prevent dopa tyrosinase reaction. As a result, there is a reduction in number, size, and aggregation of melanosomes in melanocytes and in surrounding keratinocytes. White hypopigmentation becomes more obvious as unaffected skin tans.[31,32]

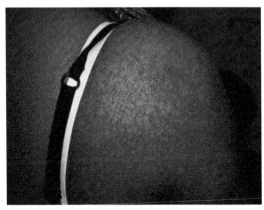

Fig. 5. Tinea versicolor. (*From* Gupta AK, Cooper EA, Simpson FC. Treatment of skin disease. Philadelphia: Elsevier, 2014; with permission.)

The upper trunk is most commonly affected, but the infection can spread to the upper arms, neck, and abdomen. Facial lesions are common in children, especially in the forehead. The eruption can itch if inflammatory but is usually asymptomatic except for skin discoloration.

Differentials of this disease include vitiligo, pityriasis alba, seborrheic dermatitis, secondary syphilis, and pityriasis rosea.

Diagnosis can be made by scraping lightly and using potassium hydroxide to examine the scale under a microscope, which should show numerous hyphae that tend to break into short, rod-shaped fragments intermixed with round spores in grape-like clusters, giving the spaghetti-and-meatballs pattern.

Topical treatment is indicated, and recurrence rates are high. Ketoconazole 2% shampoo used as a single application or daily for 3 days is highly effective and is the first choice of treatment. The shampoo should be applied to the entire skin surface from the lower posterior scalp area down to the thighs. The shampoo should be left in place for 5 minutes and then rinsed thoroughly.[33] The scalp should also be washed with shampoo at the same time. Selenium sulfide suspension 2.5% can also be applied to the entire skin surface from the lower posterior scalp down to the thighs. Using the suspension for 10 minutes every day for 7 consecutive days has resulted in an 87% cure rate at a 2-week follow-up evaluation.[34]

Terbinafine solution with spray to the affected area twice a day for 1 week is effective. Oral treatment can be used in those with extensive disease and who do not respond to conventional treatment and have frequent recurrences.

CANDIDIASIS

The yeastlike fungus *Candida albicans* and a few other Candida species are capable of producing skin, mucous membrane, and internal infections.[35] *C albicans* causes superficial infections of mucosal surface in oropharynx and genitalia in otherwise healthy individuals, whereas others manifest in setting of significant immunocompromised individuals in esophagus and tracheobronchial tree.[36]

Cutaneous candidiasis occurs on moist occluded skin, whereas disseminated candidemia occurs in immunocompromised patients.

C albicans exists as an oval yeast varying in size but has many forms such as yeast, budding yeast, pseudohyphae, and true hyphae. Antibiotic therapy increases the incidence of carriage, the number of organisms present, and the chance for tissue invasion.

Management of candidiasis includes use of oral antifungal agents, such as fluconazole tablets 50–100 to 150–200 mg or itraconazole or ketoconazole tablets. A summary of agents is provided in **Box 1**.

Cutaneous candidiasis occurs in moist, occluded cutaneous sites. It manifests with erythema, pruritus, tenderness, and pain. Cutaneous candidiasis can be found under occluded skin such as under occlusive dressing, under cast, or on the back in a hospitalized patient.

Intertrigo presents as initial pustules on an erythematous base, which becomes eroded and confluent followed by fairly sharp, demarcated polycyclic, erythematous eroded patches with small pustular lesions at the periphery (**Fig. 6**).

Diaper dermatitis presents as erythema, edema with papular and pustular lesions, erosions, oozing, and collarettelike scaling at the margins of lesions in the perigenital and perianal skin and inner aspects of thighs and buttocks. Diaper dermatitis is often treated with steroid combination creams and lotions that contain antibiotics. Dryness should be maintained by frequent changing of the diaper or leaving it off for some time.

> **Box 1**
> **Topical agents used in initial therapy for fungal vulvovaginitis**
>
> Miconazole
>
> Butoconazole
>
> Tioconazole
>
> Terconazole
>
> Clotrimazole
>
> Nystatin
>
> *Adapted from* Habif TB. Clinical dermatology: a color guide to diagnosis and therapy. Philadelphia: Mosby/Elsevier; 2004.

Antifungal creams can be applied twice a day until the eruption is clear. Mupirocin ointment, 2% applied 3 or 4 times daily, is effective for severe Candida and bacterial diaper dermatitis.

Oropharyngeal Candidiasis

Oropharyngeal candidiasis (**Fig. 7**) occurs with minor variations of host factors such as use of antibiotic therapy, use of glucocorticoid therapy, in younger and older age groups, and in those with significant immunocompromise. The etiology is one of the resident flora overgrowing in association with various local or systemic factors. Infection in the oropharynx is often asymptomatic, although a patient may have burning or pain when eating spices and acidic food, white curds on the tongue, and odynophagia. In the esophagus, it occurs when the CD4+ count is less than 200, such as in acquired immune deficiency syndrome.

Pseudomembranous candidiasis, also known as *thrush*, is a white to creamy plaque on any mucosal surface. It can vary in size from 1 to 2 mm to extensive and widespread. Removal with a dry gauze pad leaves an erythematous mucosal surface. Thrush can be found on the dorsum of tongue, buccal mucosa, hard or soft palate, the pharynx extending down into esophagus, and the tracheobronchial tree. Candidal leukoplakia are white plaques that cannot be wiped off but regress with prolonged anticandidal therapy.

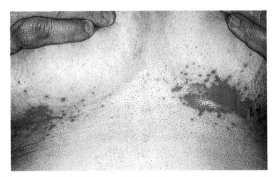

Fig. 6. Candidiasis. (*From* Habif TP, Campbell JL, Chapman MS, et al. Skin disease. 3rd edition. Philadelphia: Saunders; 2011; with permission.)

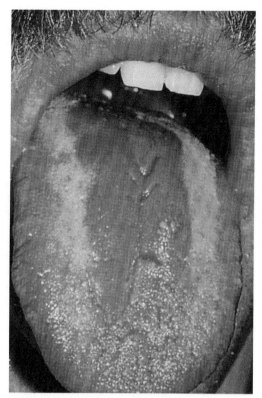

Fig. 7. Oropharyngeal candidiasis. (*From* Ignatavicius D, Workman ML. Medical-surgical nursing: patient-centered collaborative care. 8th edition. St Louis: Elsevier Saunders; 2013; with permission.)

Genital Candidiasis

Genital candidiasis occurs on nonkeratinized genital mucosa such as vulva, vagina, and preputial sac of the penis and usually represents overgrowth of endogenous colonizing *Candida* sp rather than from an exogenous source. Greater than 20% of normal women have vaginal colonization with *Candida* sp, and *C albicans* accounts for 80% to 90% of genital isolates. Risk factors include diabetes and human immunodeficiency virus/acquired immune deficiency syndrome, and pregnancy in women.[37]

Clinical manifestations include vulvitis and vulvovaginitis. Onset is abrupt, usually the week before menstruation, and symptoms include pruritis, vaginal discharge, vaginal soreness, vulvar burning, and dyspareunia. First-line therapy consists of antifungal creams as listed in **Box 1**. Oral antifungal agents include ketoconazole, fluconazole, and itraconazole. Cure rate with nystatin is 70% to 80% and with azole derivatives is 85% to 90%.[37] The initial application can cause local burning, especially if inflammation is severe. The course of treatment can be repeated if symptoms do not subside.

Candida Balanitis

The uncircumcised penis provides a warm, moist environment for yeast infections. Candida balanitis can occur after intercourse with an infected female and is more common in those who had vaginal intercourse within 3 months.[38] Tender, pinpoint, red papules and pustules appear on the glans and shaft of penis. The presence of pustules is very suggestive of candidiasis and white exudate similar to that seen in Candida vaginal infections can be present.

The eruption responds quickly to twice-a-day application for 7 days of miconazole or clotrimazole. Relief can be immediate, but treatment should last at least 7 days. A single 150-mg dose of fluconazole is comparable in efficacy and safety to clotrimazole cream applied topically for 7 days when administered to patients with balanitis.[39–41]

SUMMARY

Dermatophyte infections are common throughout the world and are most commonly caused by *Epidermophyton*, *Trichophyton*, and *Microsporum* genera. They can infect the hair, nails, beard, and different parts of the skin such as chest and groin. They can also be disguised as bacterial infections. The clinical manifestations of these fungal infections presents as tinea capitis, tinea corporis, tinea cruris, tinea pedis, and tinea barbae. An inaccurate diagnosis can lead to inappropriate treatment, such as with topical corticosteroids, which can worsen the clinical picture. Therefore, a potassium hydroxide preparation is used to confirm the diagnosis. Most of the fungal infections are treatable with topical antifungal agents and when this is ineffective, oral antifungal agents are used. It is essential for primary care providers to be aware of various presentations of dermatophyte infections and treatment options available to accurately care for their patients.

REFERENCES

1. Havlickova B, Czaika VA, Friedrich M. Epidemiological trends in skin mycoses worldwide. Mycoses 2008;51(Suppl 4):2.
2. Seebacher C, Bouchara JP, Mignon B. Updates on the epidemiology of dermatophyte infections. Mycopathologia 2008;166:335.
3. Ameen M. Epidemiology of superficial fungal infections. Clin Dermatol 2010; 28:197.
4. Crissey JT, Lang H, Parish LC. Manual of medical mycology. Cambridge (United Kingdom): Blackwell Science; 1995. p. 36.
5. Burke WA, Jones BE. A simple stain for rapid office diagnosis of fungus infection of the skin. Arch Dermatol 1984;120:1519.
6. Head ES, Henry JC, MacDonald EM. The cotton swab technique for the culture of dermatophyte infections: its efficacy and merit. J Am Acad Dermatol 1984; 11:797.
7. McBride A, Cohen BA. Tinea pedis in children. Am J Dis Child 1992;146:844.
8. Kates SG, Nordstrom KM, McGinley KJ, et al. Microbial ecology of interdigital infections of toe web spaces. J Am Acad Dermatol 1990;22:578.
9. Daniel CR, Gupta AK, Daniel MP, et al. Two feet-one hand syndrome: a retrospective multicenter survey. Int J Dermatol 1997;36:658.
10. Berman B, Ellis C, Leyden J, et al. Efficacy of a 1- week, twice-daily regimen of terbinafine 1% cream in the treatment of interdigital tinea pedis: results of placebo-controlled, double-blind, multicenter trials. J Am Acad Dermatol 1992; 26:956.
11. Savin R, De Villez RL, Elewski B, et al. One- week therapy with twice-daily butenafine 1% cream versus vehicle in the treatment of tinea pedis: a multicenter, double-blind trial. J Am Acad Dermatol 1997;36(2 Pt 1):S15.

12. Kates SG, Myung KB, McGinley KJ, et al. The antibacterial efficacy of econazole nitrate in interdigital toe web infections. J Am Acad Dermatol 1990;22:583.
13. White JE, Perkins PJ, Evans EJ. Successful 2-week treatment with terbinafine (Lamisil) for moccasin tinea pedis and tinea manuum. Br J Dermatol 1991;125:260.
14. Takama H, Nitta Y, Ikeya T, et al. Pitted keratolysis: clinical manifestations in 53 cases. Br J Dermatol 1997;137(2):282.
15. Vasquez-Lopez F, Perez-Oliva N. Mupirocine ointment for symptomatic pitted keratolysis (letter). Infection 1996;24:55.
16. Faergemann J, Mörk NJ, Haglund A, et al. A multicenter (double-blind) comparative study to assess the safety and efficacy of fluconazole and griseofulvin in the treatment of tinea corporis and tinea cruris. Br J Dermatol 1997;136:575.
17. Wharton J, Wilson P, Kincannon J. Erythrasma treated with single dose clarithromycin. Arch Dermatol 1998;134:671.
18. El-Gohary M, van Zuuren EJ, Fedorowicz Z, et al. Topical antifungal treatments for tinea cruris and tinea corporis. Cochrane Database Syst Rev 2014;(8):CD009992.
19. Van Zuuren EJ, Fedorowicz Z, El-Gohary M. Evidence-based topical treatments for tinea cruris and tinea corporis: a summary of a Cochrane systematic review. Br J Dermatol 2015;172:616.
20. Shiraki Y, Hiruma M, Hirose N, et al. A nationwide survey of Trichophyton tonsurans infection among combat sport club members in Japan using a questionnaire form and the hairbrush method. J Am Acad Dermatol 2006;54:622.
21. Bourlond A, Lachapelle JM, Aussems J, et al. Double-blind comparison of itraconazole with griseofulvin in three treatment of tinea corporis and tinea cruris. Int J Dermatol 1989;28:410.
22. Cole GW, Stricklin G. A comparison of a new oral antifungal, terbinafine, with griseofulvin as therapy for tinea corporis. Arch Dermatol 1989;125:1537.
23. Panagiotidou D, Kousidou T, Chaidemenos G, et al. A comparison of itraconazole and griseofulvin in the treatment of tinea corporis and tinea cruris: a double-blind study. J Int Med Res 1992;20:392.
24. Hubbard T. The predictive value of symptoms in diagnosing childhood tinea capitis. Arch Pediatr Adolesc Med 1999;153:1150.
25. Frieden IL. Diagnosis and management of tinea capitis. Pediatr Ann 1987;16:39.
26. Habif TP. Clinical dermatology: a color guide to diagnosis and therapy. Philadelphia: Mosby/Elsevier; 2004. p. 437.
27. Hebert AA, Head ES, MacDonald EM. Tinea capitis caused by Trichophyton tonsurans. Pediatr Dermatol 1985;2:219.
28. Gupta AK, Batra R, Bluhm R, et al. Pityriasis versicolor. Dermatol Clin 2003;21:413.
29. Nanda A, Kaur S, Bhakoo ON, et al. Pityriasis (tinea) versicolor in infancy. Pediatr Dermatol 1988;5:260.
30. Wyre HW Jr, Johnson WT. Neonatal pityriasis versicolor. Arch Dermatol 1981;117:752.
31. Galadari I, el Komy M, Mousa A, et al. Tinea versicolor: histologic and ultrastructural investigation of pigmentary changes. Int J Dermatol 1992;31:253.
32. Nazzaro-Porro M, Passi S. Identification of tyrosinase inhibitors in cultures of Pityrosporum. J Invest Dermatol 1978;71:205.
33. Lange D, Richards HM, Guarnieri J, et al. Ketoconazole 2% shampoo in the treatment of tinea versicolor: a multicenter, randomized, double-blind, placebo-controlled trial. J Am Acad Dermatol 1998;39:944.
34. Sanchez JL, Torres VM. Selenium sulfide in tinea versicolor: blood and urine levels. J Am Acad Dermatol 1984;11:238.

35. Hay RJ. The management of superficial candidiasis. J Am Acad Dermatol 1999; 40:S35.
36. Jautova J, Baloghova J, Dorko E, et al. Cutaneous candidosis in immunosuppressed patients. Folia Microbiol (Praha) 2001;46:359.
37. Fong IW. The value of treating the sexual partners of women with recurrent vaginal candidiasis with ketoconazole. Genitourin Med 1992;68:174.
38. Stary A, Soeltz-Szoets J, Ziegler C, et al. Comparison of the efficacy and safety of oral fluconazole and topical clotrimazole in patients with candida balanitis. Genitourin Med 1996;72:98.
39. Abdennader S, Casin I, Janier M, et al. Balanitis and infectious agents. A prospective study of 100 cases. Ann Dermatol Venereol 1995;122:580 [in French].
40. Elewski BE. Tinea capitis: a current perspective. J Am Acad Dermatol 2000; 42:1–20.
41. Gupta AK, Hofstader SL, Adam P, et al. Tinea capitis: an overview with emphasis on management. Pediatr Dermatol 1999;16:171.

Viral Skin Diseases

Priya Ramdass, MD[a], Sahil Mullick, MD[b],*, Harold F. Farber, MD[c]

KEYWORDS

- Exanthem • Latency • Self-limited • Enanthem • Viral shedding • Vaccination

KEY POINTS

- Viral skin diseases range from simple superficial exanthems to complex systemic diseases affecting people of all ages.
- Although not always diagnostic, the characteristic morphology, distribution, configuration, and course of the cutaneous eruptions are key components to the classification and diagnosis of viral exanthems.
- Careful assessment of infectious contacts, immunization status, and aspects of the physical examination are of considerable importance.
- Most viral exanthems are self-limited.
- Treatment, when warranted, is based on the patient's comorbidities, the extent, location, progression of the infection, and the likelihood of severe sequelae.

MEASLES (RUBEOLA)

The first scientific account of measles, differentiating it from other exanthems, is credited to the Persian physician, Muhammad Rhazes, around 900 AD.[1] It belongs to the paramyxoviridae family of the genus *morbillivirus*.[1] Measles is one of the 8 viral childhood exanthems. It is a highly contagious airborne disease that gains entry by the respiratory mucosa or conjunctiva. After an incubation period of approximately 10 days, patients begin to experience flulike symptoms with high-grade temperatures, cough, coryza, and conjunctivitis and then subsequently develop Koplik spots followed by a distinct maculopapular rash, beginning on the face and spreading cephalocaudally.[1] Although vaccination has significantly decreased the incidence of measles in developed countries, it is still prevalent in underdeveloped nations. Unsubstantiated claims suggesting that autism was linked to the measles vaccine has resulted in reduced rates of vaccination and, as a result, a resurgence of measles, mainly in unvaccinated children linked either directly or indirectly to international travel.

[a] Department of Family and Community Medicine, Mount Sinai Medical Center, 1500 South California Avenue, 10th Floor, Chicago, IL 60608, USA; [b] Department of Family Medicine, Creighton University Medical Center, 601 North 30th Street, Suite 6720, Omaha, NE 68131, USA; [c] Center for Dermatology, Laser, and Cosmetic Surgery, Psoriasis Infusion and Treatment Center, 9892 Bustleton Avenue, Suite 204, Philadelphia, PA 19115, USA
* Corresponding author.
E-mail address: Sahilmullick@creighton.edu

Prim Care Clin Office Pract 42 (2015) 517–567
http://dx.doi.org/10.1016/j.pop.2015.08.006   **primarycare.theclinics.com**

MANAGEMENT STRATEGIES
Management Goals

Measles are self-limiting, typically lasting 10 to 12 days.[2] Mainstays of treatment are supportive measures, good hydration, and primary prevention via vaccination.

Treatment Strategies

Nonpharmacologic strategies

- Increased fluid intake to prevent dehydration
- Nutritional support

Pharmacologic strategies

- Antipyretics for fever
- Vitamin A supplementation has been shown to decrease mortality and morbidity if administered daily for 2 days (**Table 1**). The mechanism of action by which this occurs is still unknown.[3]

Table 1 Vitamin A dosing recommendation	
<6 mo old	50,000 IU once daily
6–11 mo old	100,000 IU once daily
≥12 mo old	200,000 IU once daily

From Bello S, Meremikwu MM, Ejemot-Nwadiaro RI, et al. Routine vitamin A supplementation for the prevention of blindness due to measles infection in children. Cochrane Database Syst Rev 2011;(4):CD007719.

Self-Management Strategies

- Hand hygiene and airborne precaution
- Primary prevention by vaccination (refer to **Table 29**)

Evaluation, Adjustment, Recurrence

Complications

Complications most commonly include diarrhea, otitis media, predominantly in children (can lead to hearing loss), and pneumonia (most common cause of death in these patients). More serious complications include superimposed bacterial skin infections in immunosuppressed patients, hepatosplenomegaly, keratitis, encephalitis, and subacute sclerosing panencephalitis.

Recurrence

Immunity after vaccination or infection is thought to be life-long, and recurrence is rare.

EVALUATION/WORKUP
Patient History

See **Fig. 1** for an illustration of the evolution of patient symptoms.

- Atypical measles (seen in individuals vaccinated with the original killed virus from 1963 to 1967 and who have incomplete immunity) presents with subclinical prodrome symptoms and subsequently develops a rash beginning on the hands and feet and spreading centripetally.[1]

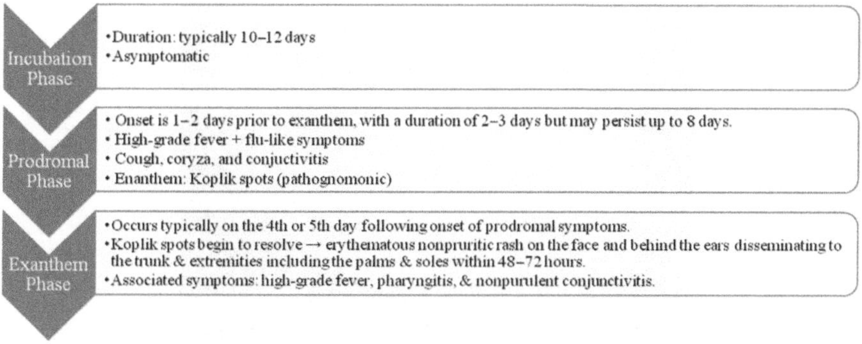

Incubation Phase	•Duration: typically 10–12 days •Asymptomatic
Prodromal Phase	• Onset is 1–2 days prior to exanthem, with a duration of 2–3 days but may persist up to 8 days. • High-grade fever + flu-like symptoms • Cough, coryza, and conjuctivitis • Enanthem: Koplik spots (pathognomonic)
Exanthem Phase	•Occurs typically on the 4th or 5th day following onset of prodromal symptoms. •Koplik spots begin to resolve → erythematous nonpruritic rash on the face and behind the ears disseminating to the trunk & extremities including the palms & soles within 48–72 hours. •Associated symptoms: high-grade fever, pharyngitis, & nonpurulent conjunctivitis.

Fig. 1. Evolution of patient symptoms. (*Data from* Kliegman RM, Nelson WE. Nelson textbook of pediatrics. Philadelphia: Elsevier Saunders; 2011; and Dietrich A, Dye LR, Hessen MT, et al. First consult. Philadelphia: Elsevier: 2015. Last updated March 11, 2015. Web. Accessed January 2, 2015.)

Physical Examination

- Prodromal phase
  - Enanthem: Koplik spots (**Fig. 2**); classically seen on the buccal mucosa, but can involve the labial mucosa and hard and soft palate
  - Nonpurulent conjunctivitis
- Exanthem phase (**Fig. 3**)
  - Exanthem: Maculopapular rash, which may begin behind the ears and face, coalesce, and within a few days, spreads to the trunk and extremities, including the palms and soles
  - Lymphadenopathy (primarily cervical) and pharyngitis
- Recovery phase: Symptoms begin to resolve 48 hours after the rash appears, and after 3 to 4 days, the exanthem darkens to a copperlike color with fine desquamation.[1,4]

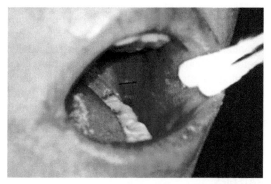

Fig. 2. Koplik spots: 1 to 3 mm grayish-white spots (resembling grains of salt) on an erythematous base. (*From* Li Z, Zhao W, Ji F. "Catarrhal physiognomy" and Koplik's spots. Braz J Infect Dis 2013;17(4):491–2; with permission.)

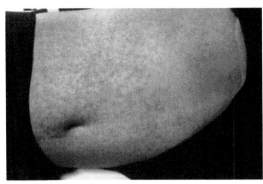

Fig. 3. Measles maculopapular erythematous blanching rash. (*From* Hirai Y, Asahata S, Ainoda Y, et al. Truncal rash in adult measles. Int J Infect Dis 2014;20:80–1; with permission.)

Imaging and Additional Testing

- Diagnosis: Koplik spots are characteristic; suspected cases can be confirmed by
  - Serology testing for antimeasles immunoglobulin M (IgM) and G (IgG) antibodies[2]
    - IgM antibodies are detectable 3 days after the exanthem appears and undetectable 1 month after the exanthem. IgG antibodies are detectable 7 to 8 days after the onset of the rash, and at least a 4-fold increase in IgG titers is confirmatory.[2,5]
  - Rapid confirmation by polymerase chain reaction (PCR) from nasopharyngeal, blood, urine, or throat specimen, which needs to be attained within 7 days of onset of the rash.[2]
  - Histologic evaluation may demonstrate keratinocytic giant cells with inclusion bodies.
- Associated laboratory findings: leukopenia, lymphocytosis, and thrombocytopenia
- Chest radiograph may reveal interstitial pneumonitis

RUBELLA (GERMAN MEASLES)

Rubella was first discovered by 2 German physicians in the 1750s.[6] It is an acquired infection that is generally benign and self-limiting. Rubella is characterized by fever, rash with lymphadenopathy, and arthritis. Preceding prodromal symptoms (seen after a 2- to 3-week incubation period) are often absent in children and mild in adults.[5] It can cause a severe congenital infection known as congenital rubella syndrome by in vitro transmission to the fetus. Although the acquired form of rubella is mild, the congenital form may have devastating effects on the fetus. The risk of developing long-term teratogenic effects of congenital infection is highest in the first trimester. With the help of mass vaccination, the incidence of acquired and congenital rubella in the United States has declined dramatically, with most cases occurring in unimmunized individuals. Rubella was officially declared nonendemic from the United States in 2004 and from the Americas in 2010.[1]

MANAGEMENT STRATEGIES
Management Goals

Management of specific congenital problems is as appropriate and with immunization.

Treatment Strategies

See **Table 2** for rubella treatment strategies.

Table 2
Rubella treatment strategies

Pharmacologic	Nonpharmacologic	Self-Management
• Antipyretics for fever • Nonsteroidal anti-inflammatory drugs for arthritis • No known effective antiviral therapy	• Supportive care • Maintain hydration • Newborn hearing and vision screen • Developmental screening • Referral to appropriate specialist	• Droplet precaution • Contact isolation to avoid contact with potentially susceptible people for 7 d after the onset of rash.[2]

Data from Romano M, Mailhot J, Wiss K. Viral exanthems: rubella, roseola, rubeola, enteroviruses. Treatment of skin disease: comprehensive therapeutic strategies. Philadelphia: Elsevier; 2013. p. 784–7.

Evaluation, Adjustment, Recurrence

Complications
Complications most commonly include joint effusions and thrombocytopenia, rarely encephalitis, spontaneous abortion and stillbirth in pregnancy, and congenital anomalies in newborns.

Recurrence
Recurrence rarely occurs because vaccination or infection typically confers life-long immunity.

Prevention
Immunization and prenatal/antepartum serologic screening, especially for women at greater risk (eg, teachers, child care employees, and health care workers), are key to prevention.

EVALUATION/WORKUP
Patient History

- Acquired infection
  - Prodrome: 1 to 5 days; low-grade fever, headache, malaise, anorexia, mild conjunctivitis, coryza, pharyngitis, cough, lymphadenopathy, and Forchheimer spots[1,5]
  - Rash (**Figs. 4** and **5**): 1 to 5 days; blotchy eruption that begins on face and neck, spreads to trunk and limbs within 24 hours, and completely resolves by the end of the third day[1,5]
- Congenital infection: Child may have mental delay and difficulty with hearing or speaking

Physical Examination

Table 3 describes the physical findings presented with acquired rubella infection and congenital rubella syndrome.

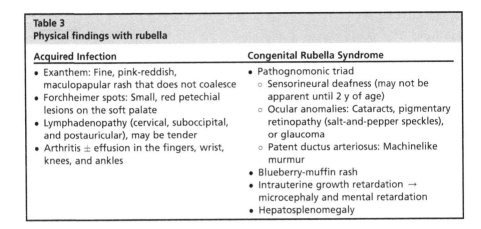

Table 3
Physical findings with rubella

Acquired Infection	Congenital Rubella Syndrome

• Exanthem: Fine, pink-reddish, maculopapular rash that does not coalesce
• Forchheimer spots: Small, red petechial lesions on the soft palate
• Lymphadenopathy (cervical, suboccipital, and postauricular), may be tender
• Arthritis ± effusion in the fingers, wrist, knees, and ankles
	• Pathognomonic triad
	  ○ Sensorineural deafness (may not be apparent until 2 y of age)
	  ○ Ocular anomalies: Cataracts, pigmentary retinopathy (salt-and-pepper speckles), or glaucoma
	  ○ Patent ductus arteriosus: Machinelike murmur
	• Blueberry-muffin rash
	• Intrauterine growth retardation → microcephaly and mental retardation
	• Hepatosplenomegaly

Imaging and Additional Testing

- Acquired infection requires confirmation by serologic testing. Enzyme-linked immunosorbent assay (ELISA; detecting either IgM or a 4-fold increase in IgG) is the diagnostic test of choice.[1]
- Congenital infection requires confirmatory testing with viral culture from nasopharynx (diagnostic method of choice) and serologic testing after 5 months of age.[1]
  - Chest radiograph is indicated in symptomatic infants.
  - Echocardiogram can be done to evaluate the severity of heart anomalies.
  - Long bone (femoral) radiograph may exhibit radiolucencies in the metaphyses.
  - Brain imaging includes intracranial calcifications, enlarged ventricles, and cortical atrophy.
- Other associated findings include leukopenia, thrombocytopenia, and increased liver function tests.

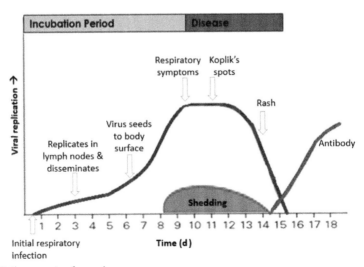

Fig. 4. Pathogenesis of measles.

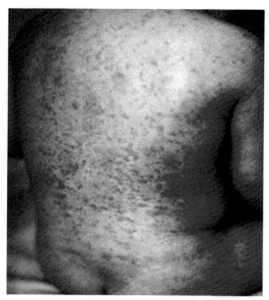

Fig. 5. Fine pink-reddish maculopapular rash of rubella that does not coalesce. (*From* the Centers for Disease Control and Prevention Public Health Image Library, ID #: 712.)

○ Cerebral spinal fluid analysis (done if rubella meningoencephalitis is suspected): leukocytes 20 to 100×10^3 with lymphocytic predominance.[1]

ERYTHEMA INFECTIOSUM (FIFTH DISEASE)

Erythema infectiosum is a contagious disease caused by parvovirus B19. Interestingly, it was discovered in 1975 during blood screening for hepatitis B (HBV) in asymptomatic donors.[7] It is most frequently seen in children between 4 and 10 years of age, but it can also affect fetuses, adults, and those who are immunocompromised.[7] Peak incidence is between late winter and early summer, often in cycles of local epidemics. Transmission occurs through exposure to droplets and fomites, person-to-person contact, and vertical and hematogenous spread. Viremia and the period of greatest infectivity occur 7 to 10 days after exposure and usually last for 1 week in immunocompetent individuals, after which time antibody production begins and the typical symptoms appear. The infection manifests as a characteristic rash in children with bilateral bright red cheeks producing the classic slapped-face appearance. In adults, the rash is less characteristic, and arthropathy is a common finding. The illness is typically transient and self-limited.[5,7]

MANAGEMENT STRATEGIES
Management Goals

- Usually, no specific treatment is indicated, and supportive therapy is sufficient.
- May need referral to specialists (cardiology, rheumatology, infectious disease, hematology, or perinatal specialist for fetal therapy).

Treatment Strategies

Table 4 describes the treatment strategies for erythema infectiosum.

Table 4		
Erythema infectiosum treatment strategies		
Pharmacologic	Nonpharmacologic	Self-Management
• Antipyretics for fever • Nonsteroidal anti-inflammatory drugs for joint symptoms • Intravenous immunoglobulin for immunocompromised patients with chronic parvovirus B19 infection and chronic anemia	• Supportive care (most cases are mild or asymptomatic and self-limited) • Screen blood products in patients with chronic hemolytic anemias, pregnancy, or immune deficiency	• Good hand hygiene • Avoid sharing food or drinks during epidemics • Once the rash develops, the child is no longer contagious and may attend school and day care

Evaluation, Adjustment, Recurrence

Complications

- Parvovirus B19 can cause fatal aplastic crisis, immune thrombocytopenic purpura, vasculitis, nephritis, lymphadenitis, meningitis, encephalitis, and fulminant liver disease.
- During pregnancy, infection with parvovirus B19 can result in fetal anemia, nonimmune hydrops fetalis, miscarriage, or fetal loss.

Recurrence
The infection generally resolves after 5 to 10 days, but can reoccur for months on exposure to sunlight, hot temperature, exercise, bathing, and stress. On complete resolution, the infection usually confers life-long immunity.[7]

EVALUATION/WORKUP
Patient History

- Rarely, individuals may also complain of fever and a painful pruritic rash on the hands and feet.
- Polyarthralgia and polyarthritis worsen throughout the day, are more commonly seen in adults (especially women), and typically involve symmetric small joints of the extremities (can be asymmetrical in children) (**Fig. 6**).

Physical Examination

- Exanthem: Classic bright red, slightly raised, nontender slapped-cheek appearance, which is often followed by a symmetric reticular, lacelike red rash on the extremities and the trunk.[5]
- Polyarthralgias and polyarthritis: edematous, slightly erythematous and tender joints.

Imaging and Additional Testing

- Clinical diagnosis
- Laboratory tests may be required for confirmation in immunosuppressed populations, those with severe anemia or transient aplastic crisis, and pregnant women
- Nucleic acid antigen testing of parvovirus B19 DNA by PCR is the most sensitive method of detection
- Associated laboratory findings: classically normocytic normochromic anemia

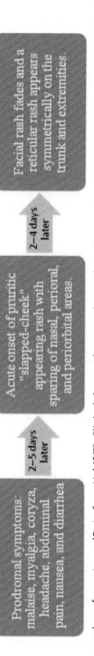

Fig. 6. Progression of symptoms. (*Data from* Habif TP. Clinical dermatology: a color guide to diagnosis and therapy. 5th edition. Philadelphia: Elsevier; 2010; and Jordan J. Clinical manifestations and diagnosis of human parvovirus B19 infection. Uptodate; 2014.)

ROSEOLA INFANTUM (SIXTH DISEASE OR ERYTHEMA SUBITUM)

Roseola infantum, also known as 3-day fever, is characterized by high-grade fever followed by abrupt defervescence and onset of a rash. It is the most common exanthem before age 2.[2] It is typically seen in children between the ages of 6 months and 4 years, with a peak age of acquisition between 9 and 21 months.[2] It is most commonly caused by human herpesvirus (HHV) -6 and less commonly by HHV-7, enterovirus, adenovirus, and parainfluenza virus.[8] The modes of transmission and incubation periods vary depending on the etiologic agent. In most patients with roseola caused by HHV-6, the average incubation period is 9 to 10 days.[8] Usually by the time the rash appears, viremia has already resolved. Recent research has shown that HHV-6 may also play a role in Kaposi sarcoma (KS), chronic fatigue syndrome, and multiple sclerosis.[8]

MANAGEMENT STRATEGIES
Management Goals

Management goals are to monitor and reduce fevers.

Treatment Strategies

Table 5 describes the treatment strategies for Roseola infantum.

Table 5		
Roseola infantum treatment strategies		
Pharmacologic	**Nonpharmacologic**	**Self-Management**
• Antipyretics for fever	• Supportive care • Adequate hydration	• Good hand hygiene • Excluded from day care if fever/rash

Evaluation, Adjustment, Recurrence

Complications
Febrile seizures, aseptic meningitis, encephalitis, and thrombocytopenic purpura.

Recurrence
Infection results in immunity.

EVALUATION AND WORKUP
Patient History

- Febrile phase: Abrupt onset of high fever (39–40°C) lasting for 3 to 5 days associated with rhinorrhea, irritability, and fatigue[2]
- Rapid defervescence followed by nonpruritic rash beginning on the trunk and then spreading to the neck, face, and proximal extremities, lasting a few hours to 3 days
- Small papules on the soft palate and uvula

Physical Examination

- Nontoxic-appearing child ± bulging fontanelles, edematous eyelids, and otitis media
- Enanthem: Nagayama spots (**Fig. 7**)[5]
- Exanthem on the trunk, neck, face, and proximal extremities (**Fig. 8**)
- Presence of cervical, postauricular, or occipital lymphadenopathy

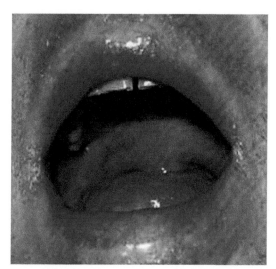

Fig. 7. Nagayama spots: erythematous papules on the soft palate and base of the uvula. (*From* Tung Y, Escutia B, Blanes M, et al. Sulfasalazine-induced hypersensitivity syndrome associated with human herpesvirus 6 reactivation and induction of antiphospholipid syndrome. Actas Dermosifiliogr 2011;102(7):537–40 [in Spanish]; with permission.)

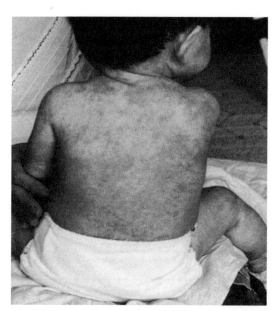

Fig. 8. Sixth disease exanthem appears as a small, pink blanching macular or maculopapular lesion surrounded by white halos. (*From* Cohen JI. Human herpesvirus types 6 and 7 (Exanthem Subitum). In: Bennett JE, Dolin R, Blaser MJ, editors. Mandell, Douglas, and Bennett's principles and practice of infectious diseases. 8th edition. Philadelphia: Saunders; 2015. *Courtesy of* Professor K. Yaminishi, Osaka University Medical School, Osaka, Japan.)

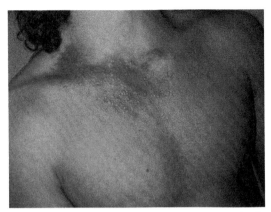

Fig. 9. Herpes simplex. (*Courtesy of* Christopher J. Huerter, MD, Chief, Division of Dermatology, Creighton Medical Center.)

Imaging and Additional Testing

- Clinical diagnosis
- Laboratory tests may be done as part of the evaluation for fever
- Associated findings: Leukocytosis and thrombocytopenia in febrile phase followed by relative neutropenia and mild atypical lymphocytosis
- Viral culture is the gold standard for confirmation but is expensive and time consuming

HERPES SIMPLEX

Herpes simplex (HSV) has 2 distinct types, type 1 and type 2, and belongs to the herpesviridae family (**Fig. 9, Table 6**).[12] HSV-1 remains the primary cause of cold sores, also known as herpes labialis, and HSV-2 is the primary cause of genital herpes.[12] HSV-1 accounts for about 20% of current cases of genital herpes in the United States.[11] Once infected, the virus lays dormant in the sensory dorsal root ganglia until it is reactivated.[10] It can be transmitted by individuals who are symptomatic or asymptomatic and even those who are unaware that they have been infected through viral shedding, and it causes painful lesions after a short incubation period. Although antivirals may help to decrease the frequency, duration, and severity of outbreaks, it is not curative.

Table 6 Comparison of herpes simplex virus-1 and herpes simplex virus-2		
	HSV-1	**HSV-2**
Transmission	Contact with bodily fluids or sexually	Sexually transmitted
Incubation	6–8 d (ranges from 1 to 26 d)[6]	4–5 d (ranges from 2 to 12 d)[6]
Pathophysiology	Oral/genital (primarily orofacial) herpes	Oral/genital (primarily genital) herpes
Latency (primary cases)	Trigeminal ganglia[10]	Lumbosacral ganglion[10]
Incidence	>70% of the population will be HSV-1 positive by 25 y old[11]	1 in every 4 individuals ≥30 y old in the United States is HSV-2-positive[11]

MANAGEMENT STRATEGIES
Management Goals

Antiviral medications can be used to reduce the severity, frequency, and duration of outbreak, with the key being to initiate therapy in the prodromal stage.

Treatment Strategies

See **Tables 7–9** for treatment strategies for HSV.

Evaluation, Adjustment, Recurrence

Complications

Disseminated HSV, encephalitis, and aseptic meningitis are severe complications. HSV-1 is associated with ocular complications (such as keratitis and acute retinal

Table 7 Pharmacologic treatment for herpes simplex virus		
	Herpes Labialis	**Genital Herpes**
Primary infection	• Anesthetic: mouth rinse with lido- caine (short-acting) or benzocaine (long-acting) • Antivirals: begin within 72 h of prodromal symptoms, for 7–10 d ○ Acyclovir: 400 mg 3 times a day (TID) or 200 mg 5 times per day ○ Famciclovir: 500 mg TID ○ Valacyclovir: 1000 mg twice daily (BID)	• Antivirals: begin within 72 h of prodro- mal symptoms for 7–10 d ○ Acyclovir: 400 mg TID or 200 mg 5 times per day ○ Famciclovir: 250 mg TID ○ Valacyclovir: 1000 mg BID • In pregnancy: Acyclovir: 400 mg TID or 200 mg 5 times per day
Recurrence	Minimal symptoms: Local anesthetics and antiseptics, no antiviral therapy is warranted • Episodic treatment: sporadic recur- rence, and well-defined prodrome ○ Acyclovir: 200 mg 5 times a day or 400 mg 3 times a day for 5 d ○ Famciclovir: 750 mg BID for 1 d or 1500 mg as a single dose ○ Valacyclovir: 2 g BID for 1 d	• Episodic treatment: <6 episodes/y or moderately symptomatic disease ○ Acyclovir: 800 mg TID for 2 d or 800 mg BID for 5 d ○ Famciclovir: 1000 mg BID for 1 d or 125 mg BID for 5 d ○ Valacyclovir: 500 mg BID for 3 d or 1000 mg daily for 5 d
	Patient should be given a supply of medication, and therapy should be initiated by the patient within 24 h of the first sign of recurrence. • Chronic suppressive therapy with acyclovir 400 mg BID or valacyclovir 500 mg daily recommended for: ○ Immunocompetent patients with ≥6 confirmed HSV episodes/y ○ Patients with systemic complica- tions (ie, erythema multiforme, eczema herpeticum, or recurrent aseptic meningitis) ○ Patients who lack a specific prodrome	• Chronic suppressive therapy: ≥6 epi- sodes per year or severely symptomatic patients ○ Acyclovir: 400 mg BID ■ Only provides suppression ■ Can be given up to 8 y without any serious adverse effects ■ In pregnancy: 400 mg TID from 36 wk gestation age till delivery ○ Valacyclovir: 500 mg daily or 1000 mg daily if >10 recurrences per year ■ Suppresses and (only antiviral that) prevents transmission ■ Can be given up to 6 y without known adverse effects ■ Foscarnet for acyclovir resistance

Data from Refs.[6,10–12]

Table 8	
Nonpharmacologic treatment for herpes simplex virus	
Herpes Labialis	**Genital Herpes**
Adequate hydration to avoid dehydration in cases with pharyngitis or gingivostomatitis	• Use sitz bath and abstain from intercourse if prodromal symptoms or lesions present • Patient education on transmission (reduced but not completely eliminated with antivirals and condom usage), course of the infection, recurrence, and preventative measures • Complete STD screening test • Delivery by cesarean section if there is the presence of prodromal symptoms or an active outbreak

Data from Refs.[6,10–12]

Table 9	
Self-management treatment strategies for herpes simplex virus	
Herpes Labialis	**Genital Herpes**
• Contact precaution (avoid contact sports, intercourse, and such) during prodromal symptoms and outbreak until lesions crust over • To prevent flare-ups in patients who have known HSV-1 and are undergoing trigeminal nerve root decompression or facial dermabrasion, consider prophylaxis antivirals	• Only high-risk patients with no history of genital lesions (ie, HIV, other STD, multiple partners, or partner with history of HSV infection) should be offered screening with type-specific serologic testing • Pregnancy: cesarean delivery is recommended if prodromal symptoms or lesions are present at the time of labor to avoid vertical transmission to neonate during vaginal delivery

Data from Refs.[6,10–12]

necrosis). HSV-2 is associated with proctitis and sacral myeloradiculitis (ie, transient urinary retention and lumbosacral sensory loss). Patients may avoid urinating due to dysuria, which may be misinterpreted as urinary retention. HSV is also associated with erythema multiforme.

- Cutaneous manifestations of HSV-1 include
  - Herpetic whitlow (**Fig. 10**) seen commonly in dentists and health care workers[6]
  - Herpetic sycosis via autoinoculation after shaving through a herpetic area[10]
  - Herpes gladiatorum, which are multiple skin lesions occurring on the face, neck, and arms in athletes participating in contact sports, such as wrestling[6]
  - Eczema herpeticum (**Fig. 11**), also known as Kaposi varicelliform eruption, which causes pain and new skin lesions in patients with atopic dermatitis, burns, or other inflammatory skin conditions[10]

Recurrence
Caused by immune-suppression, sunlight, menses, stress, trauma, trigeminal nerve manipulation, dental extractions, or genital irritation. Although frequency and severity vary, episodes of recurrence are usually shorter and milder. Genital HSV-1 recurs less frequently than HSV-2.

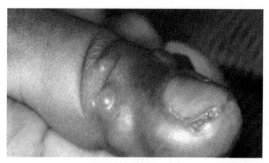

Fig. 10. Herpetic whitlow. (*From* Cohen BA. Vesiculopustular eruptions. In: Pediatric dermatology. 4th edition. Philadelphia: Elsevier; 2013. p. 104–25; with permission.)

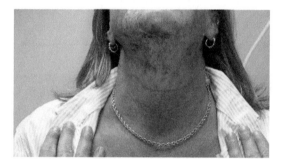

Fig. 11. Eczema herpeticum. (*Courtesy of* Christopher J. Huerter, MD, Chief, Division of Dermatology, Creighton Medical Center.)

EVALUATION/WORKUP

See **Tables 10** and **11** for signs and symptoms of herpes labilis and gential herpes, and **Figs. 12–15** for various depictions of herpes.

Table 10		
Signs and symptoms of herpes labialis		
	Patient History	**Physical Examination**
Primary infection	Prodrome: Fever, malaise, dysphagia, and pruritus → painful watery fluid-filled blisters, on vermilion border of the lip that rupture and subsequently crust → heal within 2–3 wk	Multiple clustered vesicular oral ulcers on an erythematous base in a single anatomic site ± pharyngitis or gingivostomatitis (vesiculoulcerative lesions of the oral mucosa) and regional lymphadenopathy
Recurrence	Prodrome: Pain, burning, paresthesia, and pruritus 6–48 h before vesicles → painful fluid filled blisters that rupture and subsequently crust → heal within 1 wk	Multiple clustered vesicular oral ulcers on an erythematous base in a single anatomic site +/− regional lymphadenopathy

Table 11
Signs and symptoms of genital herpes

	Patient History	Physical Examination
Primary infection (infection in a patient without antibody to HSV-1 or -2)	Prodrome: Pain at lesion site, fever, headache, malaise, dysuria, myalgia, penile/vaginal discharge	Tender vesicles and ulcers on an erythematous base in the genital area, with tender regional lymphadenopathy
Nonprimary infection (infection in patient with pre-existing HSV antibody)	Asymptomatic, subclinical, or prodrome (similar to primary infection) with moderate severity	Tender vesicles and ulcers on an erythematous base with tender regional lymphadenopathy
Recurrence (HSV type from lesion matches HSV type seen on serologic testing)	Prodrome: Ranges from mild paresthesia 30 min to 2 d before vesicle eruption to shooting pain in the gluteal area, legs or hips up to 5 d before eruption	Fewer tender vesicles and ulcers on an erythematous base with tender regional lymphadenopathy

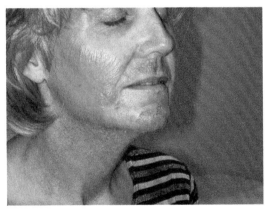

Fig. 12. Oral herpes. (*Courtesy of* Christopher J. Huerter, MD, Chief, Division of Dermatology, Creighton Medical Center.)

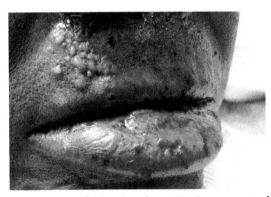

Fig. 13. Oral herpes. (*Courtesy of* Priya Ramdass, MD, Department of Family Medicine, Mount Sinai Hospital, Chicago, IL.)

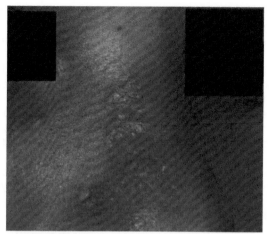

Fig. 14. HSV infection of the nose. (*From* Goodyear H. Infections and infestations of the skin. Paediatr Child Health 2015;25(2):72–7; with permission.)

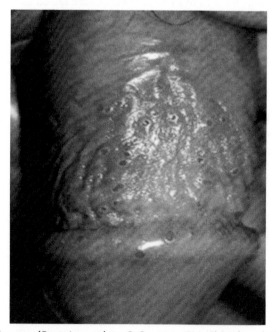

Fig. 15. Genital herpes. (*From* Leeyaphan C, Surawan TM, Chirachanakul P, et al. Clinical characteristics of hypertrophic herpes simplex genitalis and treatment outcomes of imiquimod: a retrospective observational study. Int J Infect Dis 2015;33:165–70; with permission.)

Imaging and Additional Testing

- Clinical diagnosis with confirmatory testing as the classical presentation is often absent, especially for genital herpes.
- Confirmatory tests include viral culture, PCR, direct fluorescence antibody, type-specific serologic tests.

○ Culture and PCR are the preferred methods if there are active lesions, with PCR having the greatest sensitivity and specificity.
- False-negative rate for culture sensitivity increases after 48 hours of lesion onset.
- PCR is useful for the detection of asymptomatic HSV shedding or if lesions have already crusted. However, it is costly and not routinely used.[1]

○ Serologic test
- Rapid serologic testing can be completed within 15 minutes at the primary care office and has a sensitivity and specificity of 97% and 98%, respectively.[1]
- Type-specific serologic testing is useful for diagnosis in patients with symptomatic genital disease who have healing lesions and in whom culture is likely to be negative. In addition, it may also be used in screening and can aid in the classification of infection as primary, nonprimary, or recurrent.

VARICELLA (CHICKENPOX)

Chickenpox is caused by the varicella zoster virus (VZV), which is transmitted by airborne droplets or direct contact.[10] It is typically a clinical diagnosis on the basis of the diffuse vesicular rash in various stages. The incubation period is usually 15 days, but can range from 10 to 21 days.[10] Individuals are considered highly contagious 48 hours before the characteristic exanthem appears and remain contagious until the skin lesions are fully crusted over, which occurs within 1 day, and new vesicle formation ceases (usually within 4 days).[10] Primary infection generally affects children, with more than 90% of cases occurring in children less than 10 years old, but it may also affect adults.[4] Since the unveiling of the varicella vaccine in 1995, the overall incidence of infection from VZV has significantly decreased.[4]

MANAGEMENT STRATEGIES
Management Goals

Management goals include supportive therapy and preventative measures.

Treatment Strategies

See **Table 12** for treatment strategies for VZV.

Table 12 Varicella treatment strategies	
Pharmacologic	• Acyclovir: Effective if given within the first 24 h of rash onset to: ○ Children at increased risk of complicated disease, including newborns, those with chronic skin or pulmonary disorders, those on chronic steroid therapy, or those on chronic salicylate therapy ○ Adults with uncomplicated varicella (dose: 800 mg 4 times per day for 5 d) or immunodeficiency (recommend IV acyclovir) • Varicella-zoster immune globulin indicated for VZV-exposed immune-suppressed individuals. If given within 10 d of exposure, it shortens the course of VZV but does not prevent it • Calamine lotion, pramoxine gel, or antihistamines for pruritus • Topical petrolatum or antibiotic ointments for eruptions in infants • Acetaminophen for fever (avoid aspirin in children [Reye syndrome])
Nonpharmacologic	• Airborne and contact precautions, supportive therapy, powdered baths
Self-management	Mitts and trimmed fingernails to avoid excoriation and secondary bacterial infection

Data from Refs.[1,3–5,10]

Evaluation, Adjustment, Recurrence

Complications

Complications include shingles, secondary bacterial skin infection (most common complication), hepatitis, and dehydration. Most serious complications are pneumonia, encephalitis, disseminated varicella infection, purpura, and unilateral hearing loss associated with Ramsay Hunt syndrome (typically develops insidiously within 1 week of the rash onset). In adults, pneumonia is the primary cause of morbidity and mortality, but it is rarely seen now since the introduction of the vaccine.

- In early to mid pregnancy, 1% to 2% of the fetuses may develop congenital varicella syndrome (ie, limb hypoplasia, muscle atrophy, skin scarring, microcephaly, cataracts, and rudimentary digits). If the infection occurs less than 5 days before delivery or within 2 days postpartum, the newborn is at high risk for developing disseminated varicella.[5,10]

Recurrence

Varicella infection may recur in adulthood as shingles and, in rare cases, as a milder atypical presentation with only a few papulovesicular lesions.

Prevention

Prevention is mainly through vaccination (see **Table 30**).

EVALUATION/WORKUP

Patient History

- Prodrome: Low-grade fever, malaise, anorexia, and pharyngitis occur 24 hours before the onset of the rash. Usually, children and some adults are asymptomatic before the rash.[4]
- Enanthem: Oral sores may precede the rash by 1 to 3 days or may be concurrent.[4]
- Exanthem: Diffuse, itchy, red dots resembling insect bites appear in successive crops over several days, progress over 10 to 12 hours to small bumps, blisters, and pustules, and crust over usually 1 day after the pustule appears.[4,5]

Physical Examination

- Enanthem: Small erythematous sores or blisters on the buccal surface.
- Exanthem (**Figs. 16** and **17**)
  - Stages: macule → papule → clear vesicle → pustule → crusting → healing.
  - Crusts typically slough off within 1 to 2 weeks with residual areas of hypopigmentation.[4]

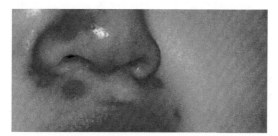

Fig. 16. Chickenpox: "dewdrop on a rose petal." (*From* Alomar MJ. Transient synovitis of the hip as a complication of chickenpox in infant: case study. Saudi Pharm J 2012;20(3):279–81; with permission.)

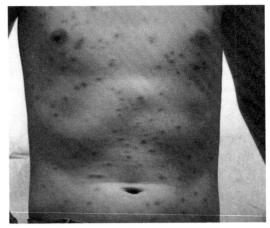

Fig. 17. Chickenpox: diffused vesicular rash surrounded by erythematous halo and eruptions in different stages. (*Courtesy of* Christopher J. Huerter, MD, Chief, Division of Dermatology, Creighton Medical Center.)

Imaging and Additional Testing

- Clinical diagnosis with chest radiograph recommended for patients with respiratory symptoms.
- Tzanck test can be used for early diagnosis.
- Even though viral culture and serologic testing are available, they are rarely done.

HERPES ZOSTER (SHINGLES)

More than one million cases of shingles occur in the United States each year, with studies depicting an increase in the incidence, associated with increasing age and decline in VZV-specific cell-mediated immunity.[5] Herpes zoster is an acute infection caused by reactivation of the latent VZV usually in the setting of a weakened immune system due to advanced age, trauma, stress, chronic diseases (such as lung, renal, inflammatory bowel disease), or immune suppression (human immunodeficiency virus [HIV] or malignancy). The risk is greater in women, Caucasians, and individuals with a family history of shingles. Zoster virus is transmitted by direct contact or inhalation of airborne droplets. Initially, the virus infects the nasopharyngeal lymphoid tissue, which leads to viremia and subsequently to chickenpox. On resolution of chickenpox, the virus remains dormant in the sensory dorsal root ganglia until it is reactivated and causes shingles. Unvaccinated persons who live to 85 years of age have a 50% risk of having zoster, and up to 3% of these people will require hospitalization.[1] Antiviral therapy is most beneficial for the elderly and the immune-compromised because it can accelerate the resolution of the lesions and decrease the severity of acute pain.

MANAGEMENT STRATEGIES
Management Goals

- Reduce the severity and duration of symptoms, prevention through vaccination
- Consider hospitalization if patient is immune-suppressed, has more than 2 dermatomes involved, has neurologic or ophthalmic involvement, or has a disseminated infection

Treatment Strategies

Nonpharmacologic treatment

- Wet compress with saline or Burow solution can help break vesicles and remove crust
- Take precautions to prevent secondary bacterial infection

Pharmacologic treatment
See **Table 13**.

Table 13 Pharmacologic treatment for shingles	

Antiviral agents	• Oral antiviral agents can be used to relieve symptoms and reduce vesicle formation if treatment is begun within 72 h of rash onset. They also help decrease the incidence of postherpetic neuralgia. Options include
	  ○ Valacyclovir 1000 mg 3 times a day for 7 d
	  ○ Famciclovir 500 mg 3 times a day for 7 d
	  ○ Acyclovir 800 mg 5 times a day for 7 to 10 d
	• Parenteral antiviral agents
	  ○ IV acyclovir is the drug of choice in cases of advanced AIDS, transplant recipient, disseminated zoster, or if there is eye involvement.
	  ○ Vidarabine is an alternative for immunocompromised patients
	  ○ Foscarnet for at least 10 d or until lesions heal if acyclovir resistance

Oral steroids	• Tapering dose of steroids (ie, prednisone starting at 40 mg/d decreased by 5 mg/d until finished) may be considered in older patients within 72 h of clinical presentation • Steroids may improve the quality of life, but they have an unfavorable risk-benefit ratio and do not prevent development of postherpetic neuralgia
Analgesics/anesthetics	• Oral: Gabapentin, tricyclic antidepressants, or narcotics • Topical: 5% lidocaine patch and capsaicin cream or patch

Data from Refs.[1,5,6]

Self-Management Strategies

- Until lesions have crusted over, patients should avoid contact with elderly or immunosuppressed persons, pregnant women, or people with no history of chickenpox and avoid scratching lesions.
- Vaccination (see **Table 30**).

Evaluation, Adjustment, Recurrence

Recurrence
Recurrence is usually induced by any type of stress.
  See **Table 14** for complications of herpes zoster.

EVALUATION/WORKUP
Patient History

Table 15 describes the symptoms of shingles.

Table 14
Complications of herpes zoster

Postherpetic neuralgia	• Pain along cutaneous nerves persisting >30 d after lesions are healed • Incidence increases with age, mainly seen in patients >60 y of age • Duration: Months or years • Treatment: Gabapentin, pregabalin, trichloroacetic acid (TCA) (eg, amitriptyline) or narcotics
Ramsay Hunt syndrome	• VZV reactivation involves the geniculate ganglion of the facial nerve • Symptoms: otalgia, vesicles on the external ear and ipsilateral oral mucosa, ipsilateral hearing loss, ipsilateral facial palsy, and vertigo ○ Ramsay Hunt syndrome may occur in the absence of a rash • Treatment: supportive, oral antivirals, steroids ± vestibular suppressants • Infectious disease consultation is recommended with close follow-up • Prognosis: fair, <50% of the cases have complete recovery of facial function
Secondary bacterial infection	• Most commonly with *Staphylococcus aureus* or *Streptococcus pyogenes*, may progress to cellulitis • Treatment: Antibiotics
Other neurologic complications	• VZV can also affect cranial nerves 2, 3, 9, and 10, causing related symptoms • Immunosuppressed persons are more prone to neurologic complications, such as encephalitis, myelitis, cranial and peripheral nerve palsies, and acute retinal necrosis
Disseminated herpes zoster (**Fig. 18**)	• More than 10 extradermatomal vesicles occurring 1–2 wk after the onset of the classic dermatomal zoster rash • Most commonly seen in immunosuppressed patients • Hospitalization is recommended
Herpes zoster oticus (**Fig. 19**)	• VZV reactivation involves the sensory ganglion of the facial nerve • Symptoms: Otalgia, vesicles on external ear ± vertigo, hearing loss, eye pain • Treatment: Oral antiviral agents and steroids • Referral to an ear, nose, and throat specialist
Herpes zoster ophthalmicus	• VZV reactivation involves the trigeminal nerve • Symptoms: Vision loss, toothache, vesicles on ipsilateral forehead and upper eyelid ○ If vesicles are noted on the tip of the nose, eye involvement is present or imminent (Hutchinson rule) • Slit-lamp examination should be done to identify corneal findings • Referral to an ophthalmologist

Data from Refs.[1,3,5,9,10]

Table 15
Symptoms of shingles

Pre-Eruptive Phase (2–3 d Before Rash Onset)	Physical Examination (Duration: 10–15 d)
• Prodrome: Fever, lassitude, headache • Pain, pruritus, and paresthesia localized to the affected dermatome region	• Patchy erythematous grouped vesicles in a beltlike pattern at various stages • Pain and pruritus

Data from Refs.[1,5,9]

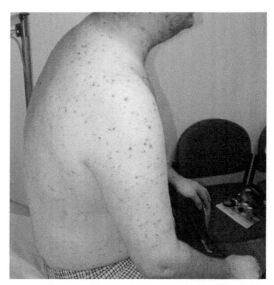

Fig. 18. Disseminated zoster: shingles. (*Courtesy of* Christopher J. Huerter, MD, Chief, Division of Dermatology, Creighton Medical Center.)

Physical Examination

- Exanthem (**Figs. 20** and **21**): ranging from macules to papules to vesicles with an erythematous base and mainly affecting the thoracic region
- Crusted lesions may resolve with or without a residual scar
- Lymphadenopathy

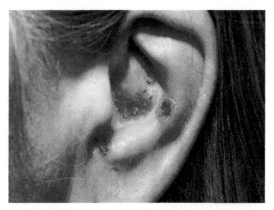

Fig. 19. Herpes zoster oticus lesions. (*From* Angles EM, Nelson SW, Higgins GL 3rd. A woman with facial weakness: a classic case of Ramsay Hunt syndrome. J Emerg Med 2013;44(1):e137–8; with permission.)

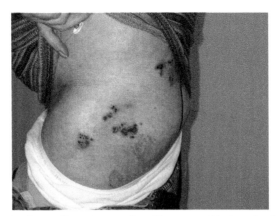

Fig. 20. Shingles: tender erythematous rash, with grouped lesions in different stages of eruption (closed, ruptured, and crusted). (*Courtesy of* Christopher J. Huerter, MD, Chief, Division of Dermatology, Creighton Medical Center.)

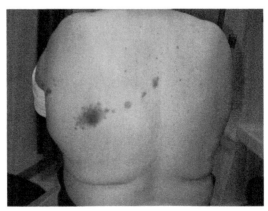

Fig. 21. Shingles contained to a dermatome in a belt-like pattern, which does not cross the midline. (*Courtesy of* Christopher J. Huerter, MD, Chief, Division of Dermatology, Creighton Medical Center.)

Imaging and Additional Testing

- Clinical diagnosis.
- Laboratory tests are generally not necessary
- PCR, viral cultures, and Tzanck test can help make the diagnosis in an atypical presentation. Samples should be obtained from vesicular fluid as crusted lesions can yield a false negative.
- Malignancy workup is not indicated in a patient with zoster. The 2 have been associated in the past, but debate exists if it is just a coincidental finding or a symptom caused by a malignant process.

KAPOSI SARCOMA–ASSOCIATED HERPESVIRUS

KS-associated herpesvirus, also known as HHV-8, is one of 7 oncoviruses (**Table 16**). Lesions from HHV-8 are described as vascular neoplasms, characterized by

Table 16
Kaposi sarcoma classification

Subtype	At-Risk Group	Cutaneous Presentation	Viscera & Lymph	Clinic Course
Classic (sporadic)	Elderly (>age 60) Males > Females, (3:1) Mediterranean and eastern European origin	Distal lower extremity	Not commonly involved	Indolent, slow-growing; rarely aggressive or diffuse; rarely affects survival
Endemic (African)	Male adults (age 20–50), children (age <10) indigenous to Africans	Adults: Local or diffuse Children: Diffuse when present; starts on face and spreads caudally	Commonly involved	Adult: Varies from nonaggressive to aggressive Children: Aggressive
Iatrogenic	Immune-suppressed (eg, solid organ transplant, medications)	Local or diffuse	Commonly involved	Often aggressive
AIDS-associated (epidemic)	Seen predominantly in homosexual men and other HIV-infected individuals	Local or diffuse	Commonly involved	This is the most aggressive type

Data from Refs[1,5,6,9,13]

inflammation, angiogenesis, and cellular proliferation. Routes of transmission include through salivary secretions, sexual transmission, blood transfusions, and organ transplant. HHV-8 is associated with KS, primary effusion lymphoma, and multicentric Castleman disease (MCD), all of which occur several years after acquiring the infection. KS is the most common tumor arising in HIV patients and is classified as an AIDS-defining illness. Individuals with increasing anti-HHV-8 antibody titers, HHV-8 viremia, HIV, poor T-cell response (immunocompromised state), and decreased levels of neutralizing antibodies are at increased risk of developing KS.[14] Although HHV-8 infection is essential for the development of KS, not all patients with HHV-8 develop the disease. Furthermore, recent studies have shown the presence of Epstein-Barr virus (EBV) DNA and β-human papilloma virus (HPV) in the lesions indicating possible coinfection.[14] Treatment varies based on the extent and location of lesions and on the progression of the disease.

MANAGEMENT STRATEGIES
Management Goals

Management goals include symptom palliation, prevent or delay disease progression, tumor shrinkage to alleviate edema and organ compromise, improve functional status, and relieve psychological stress.

Treatment Strategies

There is no gold standard of treatment of KS. Treatment is based on patient preference, comorbidities, as well as extent, location, and progression of disease (**Table 17**).

Table 17 Kaposi sarcoma treatment strategies	
Subtype	**Treatment Strategies**
Classic or endemic[15]	• Nonpharmacologic ○ Limited and asymptomatic lesions: Observation ○ Symptomatic or disfiguring lesions: Radiation, excision, cryotherapy, laser ablation ○ Compression stockings for lower extremity edema • Pharmacologic, chemotherapy if: ○ Extensive and symptomatic skill involvement or edema ○ Symptomatic visceral or mucosal involvement ○ Localized bulky disease in area that cannot be encompassed within single radiation field
Iatrogenic[5]	• Treat the cause of immune suppression and discontinue or reduce immunosuppressive medications such as corticosteroids if possible • In transplant patients, sirolimus has maintained graft function and been used to treat KS
AIDS-associated[1,5]	• Nonpharmacologic ○ Limited disease causing symptoms or cosmetic disfigurement: Intralesional chemotherapy for small lesions and radiation for larger lesions • Pharmacologic ○ Antiretroviral therapy (HAART) decreases incidence of KS and improves overall prognosis ○ Chemotherapy may be added to HAART in cases of extensive skin involvement, no response to local therapy, extensive edema, symptomatic visceral involvement, or IRIS

Data from Refs.[1,5,15]

Evaluation, Adjustment, Recurrence

Evaluation for other HHV-8-associated diseases

- Primary effusion lymphoma: Typically seen in men and boys as symptomatic serous effusion containing malignant lymphocytes without a detectable mass.[1,5] Symptoms are related to the location of fluid accumulation and include dyspnea (with pleural or pericardial effusion), ascites, joint edema, and others. It is generally resistant to chemotherapy and carries a poor prognosis.
- MCD: Classically seen in 50- to 65-year-old men with various presentations, but often presents as B symptoms (fever, night sweats, and weight loss), hepatosplenomegaly, and extensive peripheral lymphadenopathy.[1,5] There is no standard treatment, but rituximab, ganciclovir, and chemotherapy have shown promising results.

Complications associated with human herpesvirus-8 and Kaposi sarcoma treatment

- Immune reconstitution inflammatory syndrome (IRIS): Significant progression of KS within 3 months of initiating highly active antiretroviral therapy (HAART). The incidence declines with continued treatment.
- Associations of unconfirmed significance: HHV-8 DNA has been detected in several other diseases, including angiosarcoma, pemphigus vulgaris, multiple

myeloma, large plaque parapsoriasis, mycosis fungoides, idiopathic pulmonary arterial hypertension, and sarcoidosis. However, these etiologic associations have not yet been validated by studies.

Evaluation/Workup

Tables 18 and **19** describes the signs and symptoms of KS.

Table 18 Signs and symptoms of Kaposi sarcoma	
Patient History	**Physical Examination**
General symptoms: Fever, fatigue, ± B symptoms	Lymphedema in face, genitalia, and lower extremities and lymphadenopathy

• Skin lesions:
  ○ Nontender, nonpruritic lesions mainly on lower extremities and head and neck region
  ○ Violaceous papules → dark brown-black nodules
  ○ Plaquelike lesions on the soles of the feet
  ○ Varying size and morphology
  ○ Lesions may ulcerate and bleed (high vascularity)
	• Skin lesions (**Figs. 22** and **23**)
	  ○ Compressible nodules appearing fluid-filled
	  ○ Symmetric linear distribution along Langer lines
	  ○ Location: Lower extremity, sole of feet, back, face (especially nose), and genitalia
	  ○ Pigmentation: Violaceous → black nodules
	  ○ Varying sizes and shapes

• Symptoms associated with visceral organs (if involved):
  ○ Oral: Bleeding after eating, difficulty speaking, eating
  ○ GI tract (most common viscera affected and can occur without skin findings): Nausea/emesis, diarrhea, abdominal pain, malabsorption, melena, hematemesis, hematochezia
  ○ Respiratory: Dyspnea, cough, hemoptysis, chest pain
	• Symptoms associated with visceral organs:
	  ○ Oral cavity: Lesion primarily on hard palate and gingival
	  ○ GI tract: Abdominal distension, splenomegaly (immune-suppressed), tenderness on palpation, and possible signs of intestinal obstruction

Data from Refs.[5,6,9]

Table 19 Staging and prognosis of AIDS-associated Kaposi syndrome		
	Good Prognosis (Need All Listed Below)	**Poor Prognosis (Need Any Listed Below)**
Tumor (T)	T0: Confined to skin or lymph nodes and/or minimal oral disease (confined to palate)	T1: Edema or ulceration Extensive visceral KS
Immune system (I)	I0: CD4 >200/μL	I1: CD4 <200/μL
Systemic illness (S)	S0: No history of oral involvement, thrush, or other HIV-related illnesses No B symptoms Karnofsky functional score >70	S1: History of oral involvement, thrush, and/or other HIV-related illnesses (+) B symptoms Karnofsky functional score <70

Staging and prognosis are only available for AIDS-associated KS subtype.
Data from Refs.[1,5,15]

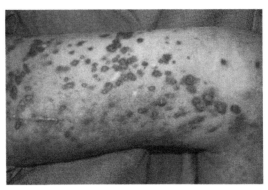

Fig. 22. Kaposi sarcoma. Multiple violaceous to hyperpigmented patches and plaques with AIDS. (*From* Brinster NK, Liu V, A. Diwan AH, et al. Dermatopathology: high-yield pathology. Philadelphia: Elsevier, 2011; with permission.)

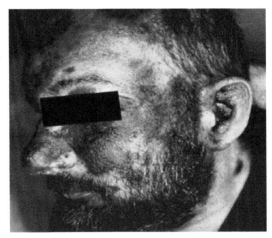

Fig. 23. Kaposi sarcoma—large confluent hyperpigmented patch stage lesions with lymphedema. (*From* Vaccher E, Tirelli U. Neoplastic disease. In: Cohen J, Powderly WG, editors. Infectious diseases, 3rd edition. St. Louis, Mosby, 2010; with permission.)

Imaging and Additional Testing

- CD-4 count and HIV viral load are essential for staging and prognosis. CD-4 count is the most important factor associated with the development of KS.
- Computed tomographic chest/abdomen/pelvis scan for staging and evaluation and endoscopic screening are not indicated in asymptomatic patients. The following diagnostic tests can be considered if visceral involvement is suspected:
  - Gastrointestinal (GI): Fecal occult blood, if positive → upper endoscopy(hemorrhagic nodules are seen)
  - Respiratory: Chest radiograph (findings vary) → if suspicious lesion → bronchoscopy (characteristic finding: cherry red lesions)
- Biopsy (preferably lymph node) with PCR or latent associated nuclear antigen by immunohistochemistry is required to identify HHV-8 DNA and confirm the diagnosis.

WARTS (VERRUCA)

The HPV is the highly contagious culprit associated with the development of warts. It is transmitted by direct contact, which causes viral infection of the epidermis.[16] Currently, there are 120 types identified and circulating in the human population today. Of all the various types of warts, genital warts, also known as condyloma acuminatum, is the only wart that is considered a sexually transmittable disease.[16] The incubation period varies and can range from 3 weeks to 8 months. Before developing the wart, most people have vague prodromal signs, such as itching and burning. After an initial outbreak, the virus remains in the body and poses the possibility of recurrence. Presently, there is no cure for HPV. Even though most warts normally resolve on their own with time, various treatment options are available for those who choose more aggressive management, and preventative measures should always be taken to reduce the likelihood of transmission.

MANAGEMENT STRATEGIES
Management Goals

- Observation is an option because some types of warts can spontaneously regress within 1 to 2 years. However, it is easier to treat fewer and smaller warts early on. Three major treatment options are chemical or physical obliteration, immunologic therapy, and surgical excision.[5]
- If there is no response to the initial therapy after 3 weeks or complete resolution has not occurred by 12 weeks, it is appropriate to switch to a different method.[5]

Treatment Strategies

Table 20 explains treatment strategies for warts.

Self-Management Strategies

- Avoid using tools, such as nail file, pumice stone, and so on, on normal skin or nails to trim warts.
- Duct tape use as an adjunct to salicylic acid therapy is uncertain.
- For plantar warts, wear protective footwear in bathhouses, communal changing rooms, and showers.

Evaluation, Adjustment, Recurrence
Complications

Genital warts can occasionally develop into large exophytic masses than can interfere with defecation, vaginal delivery, and intercourse. If it involves the proximal anal canal, it can cause strictures.

Complications associated with treatment include larger lesions can form keloids with destructive modalities, and care needs to be taken when deciding on therapy. If care is not taken with procedures such as cryosurgery, destruction to the nail matrix causing permanent damage to nail or nerve damage can occur.

- **Tables 21–23** describe diseases associated with HPV.
- Other association: Verrucous carcinoma is a low-grade, well-differentiated form of SCC. It is thought to be associated with both high- and low-risk genotypes. It can be divided into 3 distinct clinicopathologic types based on anatomic area of involvement: oral florid papillomatosis (oral cavity), giant condyloma of Buschke and Löwenstein (anogenital area), and carcinoma cuniculatum (palmoplantar surface). These tumors rarely metastasize.

Table 20 Treatment strategies for warts	
Wart	**Treatment Strategies**
Verruca vulgaris (common wart) Verruca plantaris (plantar wart)	• Pharmacologic: Salicylic acid ○ Treatment of choice for children and dark-skinned individuals • Nonpharmacologic: Cryotherapy ○ Treatment of choice for light-skinned individuals
Verruca plana (flat wart)	• Pharmacologic: 5-fluorouracil or imiquimod ○ Treatment of choice for dark-skinned individuals • Nonpharmacologic: cryotherapy ○ Treatment of choice for light-skinned individuals
Condyloma acuminatum (genital wart)	• Pharmacologic: ○ Nonpregnant women with restricted vulvar disease capable of self-treatment: Imiquimod ○ Nonpregnant women with restricted vulvar disease who are not capable of or fail self-therapy, or pregnant women with symptomatic warts: TCA ○ Nonpregnant women with restricted vulvar disease that does not resolve with monotherapy: Imiquimod + TCA • Nonpharmacologic: ○ Laser ablation is the preferred surgical approach if size >20 cm^2 and/or bulky disease ○ Anoscopy and vaginal speculum examination (if applicable) should be done to evaluate the extent of disease
Periungal (nail) wart	Laser therapy has been proven to be effective, whereas cryosurgery and salicylic acid treatments are not due to the location of the wart
Filiform (digitate) wart	Treatment method of choice is snip or shave excision

Data from Refs.[5,6,10,16–18]

Recurrence

The virus may still be present in remaining tissue after a successful treatment, which can cause recurrence.

- On recurrence, either excisional or fulguration therapy is recommended to obtain a specimen for analysis. Approximately 4 weeks after the procedure, when the area is healed, imiquimod cream is used as adjuvant treatment for 12 weeks.[6]

Table 21 Nongenital cutaneous disease	
Association	**HPV Type**
Ungal squamous cell carcinoma	HPV 16
Epidermodysplasia verruciformis	Known as "tree man illness." Rare autosomal-recessive skin disorder associated with more than 15 types of HPV; results in lifelong eruptions of pityriasis versicolor-like macules, flat wart-like papules, and development of cutaneous carcinomas
Butcher's warts	Common warts on the hands of people who handle meat, poultry, and fish; caused by HPV 1–4, 7, 10, and 28

Data from Refs.[5,6,10,16,17]

Table 22
Nongenital mucosal disease

Association	HPV Type
Respiratory and laryngeal papillomatosis	HPV 6 and 11
Laryngeal carcinoma	HPV 6 and 11
Maxillary sinus papilloma	HPV 57
Conjunctival carcinoma	HPV 16
Oropharyngeal cancer	HPV 16
Heck disease	Also known as focal epithelial hyperplasia; white-pinkish papules occur diffusely in the oral cavity; HPV 13 and 32

Data from Refs.[5,6,10,16,17]

Table 23
Anogenital disease

Complication	HPV Type (Mainly High-Risk HPV 16 and 18)
Cervical disease	Low-grade squamous intraepithelial lesion or high-grade squamous intraepithelial lesion → cervical cancer
Vulvar and vaginal cancer	Vulvar cancer also associated with HPV 6 and 11
Penile cancer	—
Anal cancer	Most commonly causes SCC; also associated with HPV 31–33
Bowenoid papulosis	Pigmented verrucous papules on the penis
Bowen disease	Associated with varies types of HPV but mainly 16

Data from Refs.[5,6,10,16–18]

Prevention

- Vaccination (see **Table 31**)[19]
- Plantar warts: Patients should keep their feet clean and dry and wear protective footwear in communal bathing or changing areas.
- Periungal wart: Patients should not bite or pick at their nails.

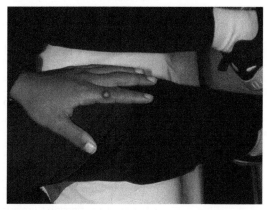

Fig. 24. Verruca vulgaris. (*Courtesy of* Christopher J. Huerter, MD, Chief, Division of Dermatology, Creighton Medical Center.)

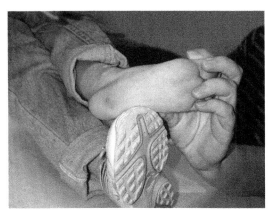

Fig. 25. Verruca plantaris. (*Courtesy of* Christopher J. Huerter, MD, Chief, Division of Dermatology, Creighton Medical Center.)

EVALUATION AND WORKUP
Patient History and Physical Examination

See **Table 24** for signs and symptoms of warts.

Table 24 Signs and symptoms of warts	
Lesion	**Signs and Symptoms**
Verruca vulgaris (common wart) (**Fig. 24**)	• Location: Mainly hands but can occur anywhere • Painless, raised, rough, and dome shaped • Skin colored • Size: Ranges from the size of a pinhead to 10 mm
Verruca plantaris (plantar wart) (**Fig. 25**)	• Location: Pressure points on the soles of the feet • Pain with walking described as "walking on a stone" • Appearance: Varies from a hard, small, black, punctate lesion to a brownish, rough, firm, well-demarcated lesion with pinpoint black spot or spots due to clotted blood vessels
Verruca plana (flat wart)	• Location: Mainly face, forehead, and areas frequently shaved • Painless, slightly raised above the skin, smooth, and flat topped • Skin colored, light brown or yellow • Size: Size of a pinhead and hundreds clustered in one location
Condyloma acuminatum (genital wart) (**Fig. 26**)	• Location: Genitals • Raised and resembling a cauliflower • Flesh colored or whitish-gray
Periungal wart (nail wart)	• Location: Adjacent to or on the cuticle • Size varies from a pinhead, raised, smooth, with uneven borders to pea-sized, rough, and irregularly shaped • Can affect nail growth and nail elevation
Filiform wart	• Location: Face (mainly near eyelids and lips) • Narrow, long, fingerlike projections that may be single or in clusters, flesh-colored

Imaging and Additional Testing

- Most cutaneous and external genital warts are diagnosed by clinical examination or with application of acetic acid and biopsy. If a wart has been chemically treated and a subsequent biopsy is done, the pathologist should be notified because it may resemble an anaplastic lesion.
- Papanicolaou test ± HPV testing to screen for cervical neoplasia based on guidelines for cervical cancer screening and colposcopy if needed.
- Consider screening for other sexually transmitted infections.

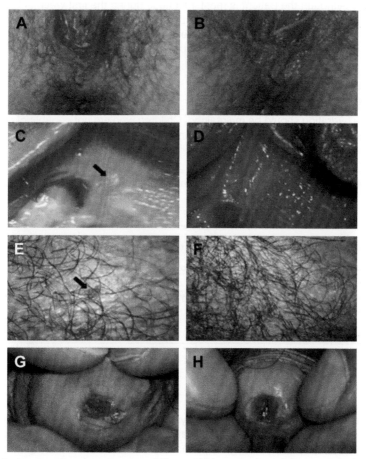

Fig. 26. Pretreatment and posttreatment (1 month) images of condylomata acuminata with topical photodynamic therapy. (*A*), (*C*), (*E*), (*G*) Show condyloma's prior to treatment. (*B*), (*D*), (*F*), (*H*) Shows the same area 1 month after treatment with topical photodynamic therapy. (*From* Nucci V, Torchia D, Cappugi P. Treatment of anogenital condylomata acuminata with topical photodynamic therapy: report of 14 cases and review. Int J Infect Dis 2010;14 Suppl 3:e280–2; with permission.)

HAND, FOOT, AND MOUTH DISEASE

Hand, foot, and mouth disease is one of most easily recognized viral exanthem in childhood. It was first described in 1957 after a summer outbreak in Toronto,

Canada.[20] It is a highly contagious disease, most commonly caused by coxsackievirus A16 followed by enteroviruses.[10] Although it primarily affects children less than 10 years of age, it can also affect adults. Children less than 5 years of age are at higher risk of infection.[4] Enterovirus infections are more common in Asia and are known to be more severe and even fatal.[20] The virus is transmitted through direct contact with bodily fluids or by the fecal-oral route, as both viruses proliferate in the intestinal tract and are found in pharyngeal secretion and stool. On average, symptoms develop 3 to 5 days after exposure and include low-grade fever, herpangina, and rash on the feet, hands, extremities, and buttocks. Complete resolution typically occurs within 7 to 10 days.[10] Although the patient is most infectious during the first week of the illness, he or she can still be contagious after symptoms have resolved because the virus remains in the body for approximately 6 weeks.[20] Currently, studies are being done to develop a vaccine or antiviral agent to help prevent and treat the infection.[20]

MANAGEMENT STRATEGIES
Management Goals

Adequate hydration should be maintained. Children who are not capable of tolerating oral intake should be hospitalized for parenteral fluids.

Treatment Strategies

See **Table 25** for treatment strategies for hand, foot, and mouth disease.

Table 25 Hand, foot, and mouth disease treatment strategies		
Pharmacologic	**Nonpharmacologic**	**Self-Management**
• Antipyretics for fever • Topical oral anesthetics for painful oral ulcers	• Supportive care • Maintain hydration	• Contact precaution • Exclusion from day care/school if skin lesions are present • Good hand hygiene • Disinfect surfaces and fomites

Evaluation, Adjustment, Recurrence

Complications
Complications include dehydration, nail dystrophy, and onychomadesis. Enterovirus is associated with more serious complications, including rhombencephalitis, acute flaccid paralysis, aseptic meningitis, pulmonary edema and hemorrhage, and heart failure.

Recurrence
Immunity is established after infection, but a second episode can occur if infected by a different virus.

EVALUATION/WORKUP
Patient History

- Possible exposure history: Day care, play area, public swimming area, or exposure to treated waste water or sick contact within the past month (**Fig. 27**)

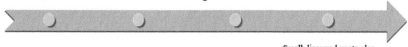

Prodromal symptoms (irritability, emesis, diarrhea, and abdominal pain) are typically absent but, if present, appear 4–6 days after incubation

Dysphagia or refusal to eat (in non verbal children) due to painful red oral lesions on the tongue or buccal mucosa.

Low-grade fever

Small dispersed nontender non pruritic blisters, with red halos on the hands, feet, extremities, and buttocks

Fig. 27. Progression of symptoms. (*Data from* Romero JR. Hand, foot, and mouth disease and herpangina: an overview. Uptodate; 2014.)

Physical Examination

- Lymphadenopathy
- Infection with enterovirus should be considered if patient develops tachycardia, tachypnea, and cyanosis, usually 1 to 3 days after symptom onset (**Fig. 28**)[5]

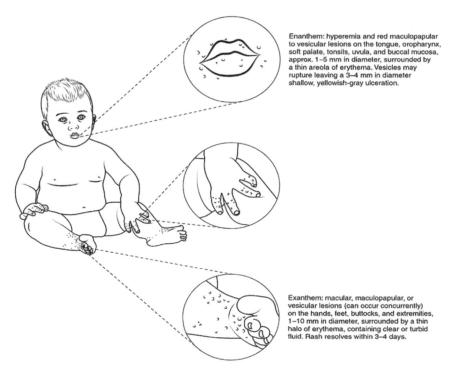

Enanthem: hyperemia and red maculopapular to vesicular lesions on the tongue, oropharynx, soft palate, tonsils, uvula, and buccal mucosa, approx. 1–5 mm in diameter, surrounded by a thin areola of erythema. Vesicles may rupture leaving a 3–4 mm in diameter shallow, yellowish-gray ulceration.

Exanthem: macular, maculopapular, or vesicular lesions (can occur concurrently) on the hands, feet, buttocks, and extremities, 1–10 mm in diameter, surrounded by a thin halo of erythema, containing clear or turbid fluid. Rash resolves within 3–4 days.

Fig. 28. Classic findings associated with hand, foot, mouth disease.

Imaging and Additional Testing

- Primarily a clinical diagnosis
- Confirmation of a specific viral cause is not warranted in children with uncomplicated course. If confirmation is needed, real-time-PCR or nucleic acid amplification from vesicular fluid is the diagnostic method of choice. Cell cultures may be done but are less sensitive then the aforementioned tests.
- Blood, throat, and stool samples are less useful because isolation and identification of the virus is time-sensitive, especially in cases of enterovirus infection, and do not conclusively establish causality.
- Associated nonspecific laboratory findings include hyperglycemia and neutrophilia.

MOLLUSCUM CONTAGIOSUM

Molluscum contagiosum is caused by the molluscum virus (which is part of the poxvirus family) with the only known host being humans. Four distinct genotypes have been identified, with genotype 1 being the predominant type that causes 90% of the cases in the United States.[21] In recent years, there has been a gradual increase in the number of cases in healthy children, adults with sexually transmitted diseases (STD), and immunocompromised patients.[5] The virus is transmitted through direct skin contact, including sexual activity, contact sports, contact with fomites, or autoinoculation by scratching or touching an infected lesion. Lesions characterized by grouped, dome-shaped papule with an umbilicated center, often appear around 7 weeks after exposure, are extremely contagious and remain so until the papules have completely resolved. It commonly affects the face, trunk, axillae, and extremities in children and the pubic and genital areas in adults. If genital lesions are present, it is considered a STD, and in the case of children, sexual abuse should be suspected. In healthy individuals, lesions are rarely severe as the virus only affects the outer (epithelial) layer of the skin.[21] Lesions spontaneously resolve within 2 months, often clearing completely within 6 to 12 months without treatment and without scars.[5] However, patients with immunosuppression (ie, HIV), atopic dermatitis, or other skin diseases may have a more extensive presentation.[5]

MANAGEMENT STRATEGIES
Management Goals

Full skin examination is imperative because incomplete treatment may result in continued autoinoculation and failure cure. The infection is self-limited in immunocompetent individuals, and treatment in such cases is optional, especially if it involves children or pregnant patients. Individuals with genital lesions and those who are immunosuppressed should be treated to prevent spread and reduce disease severity. Repeat examination is recommended 2 to 4 weeks after treatment.[21]

Treatment Strategies

When a trial of treatment is desired, cryotherapy, curettage, podophyllotoxin, or cantharidin are considered first-line options based on the rapid, clinically evident response associated with their use. Conservative, nonscarring methods should be used for people with multiple lesions (**Table 26**).

Evaluation, Adjustment, Recurrence

Complications
Complications include bacterial superinfection and follicular or papillary conjunctivitis (if on the eyelid).

Recurrence
Reinfection may occur on exposure to an infected person.

EVALUATION AND WORKUP
Patient History

- Usually painless, smooth, firm, dome-shaped lesions with a dimple or pit in the center. May be associated with local erythema, swelling, and pruritus
- Most commonly on the trunk, axillae, crural folds, and antecubital and popliteal fossae
- Spares the oral mucosa, palms, and soles

Table 26
Molluscum contagiosum treatment strategies

Pharmacologic	• Cantharidin: Preferably applied by a physician to prevent inadvertent spread of the vesicant to other areas. Once applied, it remains on for 2–6 h or until the first signs of blistering and then is washed off with soap and water. Avoid applying on the face and genital and perianal areas
	  ○ Usual course of each treatment requires 2 visits to achieve complete clearance. Treatment can be repeated every 2–4 wk until all lesions have resolved. With proper application, lesions resolve without scarring
	  ○ Common adverse effects: Transient burning, pain, erythema, and pruritus at application site. Postinflammatory dyspigmentation may occur, but it topically resolves over several months
	• Podophyllotoxin: Self-applied twice a day for 3 wk and used for infectious lesions on the thighs or genitalia
	  ○ Adverse effect: Local erythema, burning, pruritus, inflammation, erosion
	  ○ The safety and efficacy in young children is not definitively established
	• Other agents: Imiquimod, potassium hydroxide, salicylic acid, topical retinoids, and oral cimetidine have also been used for the treatment of lesions. However, there are insufficient data in support of the efficacy of these treatments. Use of retinoids is contraindicated in pregnancy

Nonpharmacologic	• Cryotherapy: In-office procedure and rapidly effective. This conservative method destroys most lesions in 1 to 3 treatment sessions at 1- or 2-wk intervals and rarely produces a scar, making it first-line treatment for many clinicians. Most children will not tolerate cryotherapy due to the pain associated with the procedure • Curettage: Useful when there are a few lesions because it provides the quickest, most reliable treatment. Topical anesthesia may be needed when treating children. A small scar may form; thus refrain from applying in cosmetically important areas • Other: Hypoallergenic surgical adhesive tape and laser therapy
Self-Management	• Contact precaution: Not necessary to remove children from day care or school or to exclude from playing contact sports provided that the lesions are properly covered with clothing or dressing. Bathing with other children should be avoided • Efficacy of condoms preventing spread is unclear; abstinence should be encouraged until resolution • Sharing towels, clothing, or other personal items should be discouraged • Shaving the area around the lesion should be discouraged

- Sexually transmitted molluscum contagiosum involves the groin, genitals, proximal thighs, and lower abdomen

Physical Examination

- Exanthem (**Figs. 29** and **30**): Dome-shaped papules, slightly umbilicated with a caseous plug, with or without surrounding inflammation (presence is a sign of impending regression)
- Conjunctivitis if the lesion is located on the eyelid
- Molluscum dermatitis (**Fig. 31**): Development of eczematous patches or plaques surrounding molluscum lesions
- Papules may be large, multiple, and widespread in HIV or immune-suppressed patients

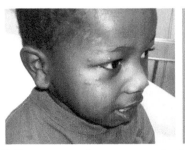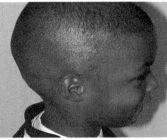

Fig. 29. Molluscum contagiosum seen on the face and scalp of a child. Flesh-colored, dome-shaped papules. (*Courtesy of* Christopher J. Huerter, MD, Chief, Division of Dermatology, Creighton Medical Center.)

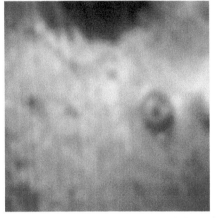

Fig. 30. Molluscum contagiosum: discrete 2- to 5-mm, slightly umbilicated, flesh-colored, dome-shaped papules with a caseous plug. (*From* Peterson BW, Damon IK. Other poxviruses that infect humans. In: Bennett JE, Dolin R, Blaser MJ, editors. Mandell, Douglas, and Bennett's principles and practice of infectious disease. 8th edition. Philadelphia: Saunders; 2015. p. 1703–6; with permission.)

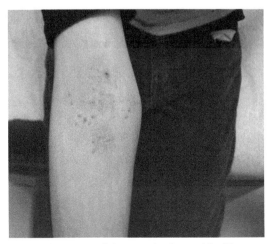

Fig. 31. Molluscum contagiosum overlying atopic dermatitis. (*Courtesy of* Christopher J. Huerter, MD, Chief, Division of Dermatology, Creighton Medical Center.)

Imaging and Additional Testing

- Mainly a clinical diagnosis
- If necessary, rapid confirmation can be made by removing a small lesion with a curette and placing it with a drop of potassium hydroxide between 2 microscope slides. The preparation is gently heated and then crushed with firm, twisting pressure. The content of the papule that contains infected cells can be examined directly in a heated potassium hydroxide preparation. The infected cells are dark and round and disperse easily with slight pressure, whereas normal epithelial cells are flat and rectangular and tend to remain stuck together in sheets.
- Individuals with greater than 20 to 30 lesions should be examined for underlying diseases such as STD, HIV, or malignancy.[21]

GIANOTTI-CROSTI SYNDROME

Gianotti-Crosti syndrome (GCS) is an acute onset of symmetric, erythematous, papular eruptions that are accentuated on the face, extensor surfaces of the extremities, and the buttocks. It often presents with lymphadenopathy and anicteric hepatomegaly. It most commonly occurs in children between the ages of 1 and 3 years, but may occur in older children, adolescents, or adults. In childhood, both sexes are equally affected; however, in adulthood, women are more prone to developing GCS than men. The exanthem can last anywhere from 2 weeks to 6 months, but typically resolves within 2 to 8 weeks.[5]

Since the discovery of GCS in the 1950s, several viruses have been associated with its cause. HBV and EBV are the predominant culprits, with EBV being the most common cause in the United States due to routine HBV vaccination in infants. Originally, GCS had 3 cardinal manifestations[10]:

- Nonrelapsing erythematopapular dermatitis localized to the face and limbs, lasting about 3 weeks[10]
- Paracortical hyperplasia of lymph nodes[10]
- Acute hepatitis, often anicteric, can last for months and progress to chronic liver disease[10]

However, with current terminology, neither lymphadenopathy nor hepatitis is required for the diagnosis of GCS. Because of its benign and self-limited nature, most cases are either not reported or often misdiagnosed as a nonspecific viral exanthem. Diagnostic testing is only done for viral confirmation in cases of immune suppression or pregnancy.

MANAGEMENT STRATEGIES
Management Goals

Benign, self-limited disease; lesions usually clear within 4 to 12 weeks[1]

Treatment Strategies

See **Table 27** for GCS treatment strategies.

Table 27
Gianotti-Crosti syndrome treatment strategies

Pharmacologic	Nonpharmacologic	Self-Management
• Antihistamine or calamine lotion for pruritus	• Supportive care • Adequate hydration	• Exclusion from day care or school is not necessary

Evaluation, Adjustment, Recurrence

- For GCS due to HBV infection, regular follow-up and liver function test monitoring are recommended. If the alanine aminotransferase level remains elevated for more than 6 months, it indicates chronic hepatitis, and the patient should be referred to a gastroenterologist, hepatologist, or an infectious disease specialist.[1]
- Complications: Acute HBV infection may progress to chronic infection.
- Recurrence: Possible but rare.

EVALUATION AND WORKUP
Patient History

- Upper respiratory or GI illness 1 week before the onset of the exanthem
- Sudden onset of a symmetric rash starting on the lower extremities and ascending upwards to involve the buttocks, upper arms, and face within 3 to 4 days
- Associated symptoms: Pruritus, malaise, low-grade fever, or diarrhea

Physical Examination

- Exanthem (**Fig. 32**): Symmetric, flat, papular, or papulovesicular rash on the extensor surfaces of the extremities, buttocks, or face with sparing of the trunk and mucosal surfaces. Rash can coalesce into larger plaques
- Lymphadenopathy: Cervical, axillary, or inguinal
- Anicteric hepatomegaly

Imaging and Additional Testing

- Clinical diagnosis
- Nonspecific laboratory findings include elevated liver enzymes, lactate dehydrogenase, and alkaline phosphatase without hyperbilirubinemia
- If due to HBV, (+)HBV surface antigen
- Skin biopsy cannot confirm the diagnosis, but it may be necessary to exclude other differential diagnoses if the rash is atypical

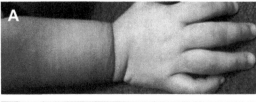
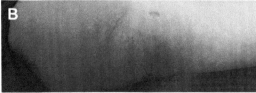

Fig. 32. (*A–B*) Monomorphous, symmetric, flat-topped, lichenoid, flesh-colored to reddish-brown papules or papulovesicles, 3 to 4 mm in diameter. (*From* AlSabbagh MM, Hussein Kassim AK. Gianotti–Crosti syndrome—the first case report from Bahrain: a rare presentation following vaccinations. J Dermatol 2015:19(2); with permission.)

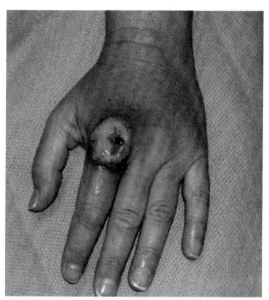

Fig. 33. Orf bullae. (*Courtesy of* Christopher J. Huerter, MD, Chief, Division of Dermatology, Creighton Medical Center.)

ORF (CONTAGIOUS ECTHYMA)

Orf is a zoonotic viral disease caused by the parapoxvirus orf virus and is commonly seen in veterinarians, farmers, shepherds, butchers, and meat porters. Those infected with this virus initially appear well, with only a low-grade fever, followed by development of a tender small papule on the hand or finger or fingers, that progressively enlarges to a blister (shown in **Fig. 33**), approximately 1 week after direct contact with an infected animal (primarily sheep or goat), animal products, or contaminated fomite (**Figs. 33** and **34**). Shortly after the blister ruptures, the lesion resolves without any scarring (See **Fig. 34**). Although it is more prevalent in Europe and New Zealand, there

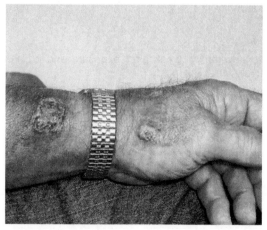

Fig. 34. Orf—ecthyma contagiosum. (*Courtesy of* Christopher J. Huerter, MD, Chief, Division of Dermatology, Creighton Medical Center.)

have been cases reported in North America. Because of its commonality among farmers, veterinarians, and shepherds, and given the benign self-limited nature of the disease, cases are not reported as frequently. Barrier protection and proper hand hygiene are strongly recommended to help reduce the likelihood of transmission.

MANAGEMENT STRATEGIES
Management Goals

Benign, self-limited with complete resolution within 1 month after onset

Treatment Strategies

See **Table 28** for Orf treatment strategies.

Table 28
Orf treatment strategies

Pharmacologic	Nonpharmacologic	Self-Management
• Cidofovir • Imiquimod Both medications have shown promising results but lack clinical data depicting their efficacy	• Moist dressings • Local antiseptics • Finger immobilization • Surgical care (curettage or electrodessication) for large exophytic or persistent lesions	• Barrier protection (ie, gloves) • Hand hygiene

Evaluation, Adjustment, Recurrence

Complication
Secondary bacterial infection, toxic erythema.

Recurrence
Can occur but lesions are less pronounced than the primary infection.

EVALUATION/WORKUP
Patient History

- Low-grade fever with subsequent development of a tender nodule on the hand or finger or fingers.

Physical Examination

- Tender nodule develops 1 week after exposure and progresses through the stages, as shown in **Fig. 35**.

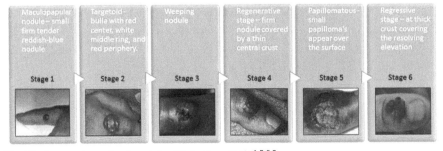

Fig. 35. Progression of orf nodule. (*Data from* Refs.[1,5,6,9])

- Regional lymphadenopathy or adenitis may also be present.

Imaging and Additional Testing

- Clinical diagnosis; serologic tests are not routinely required.
- Real-time PCR is the diagnostic test of choice to confirm a clinic diagnosis.
- Electron microscopy can be used, but it lacks the ability to distinguish between the various parapoxviruses.

MONKEYPOX

The first human infection with Monkeypox virus was identified in western and central Africa in the 1970s. The first outbreak in the western hemisphere occurred in the United States in 2003. Monkeypox is a zoonotic infection that is acquired through respiratory contact or direct contact with the infected animal's body fluids, skin lesions, or contaminated fomites. It belongs to the same genus as variola virus (the causative agent of smallpox) and vaccinia virus (the virus used in the smallpox vaccine). The pathogenesis of human monkeypox is similar to that of smallpox except monkeypox is associated with a greater degree of lymphadenopathy and lower capacity for person to person transmission. During the incubation period of 4 to 20 days, the virus is delivered to the internal organs and the skin. Subsequently, patients begin to experience flulike symptoms followed by an exanthem involving the palms and soles.[9] The illness lasts 2 to 4 weeks and then resolves.[22] Patients are considered contagious until the crusts on the lesions are shed.

MANAGEMENT STRATEGIES
Management Goals

Self-limited; mainly supportive, with case-to-case spread reduced through isolation, and, if available, the use of smallpox vaccine for contacts

Treatment Strategies
Nonpharmacologic strategies

- Supportive therapy including adequate hydration and bed rest

Pharmacologic strategies

- Currently no antiviral drugs are licensed to treat orthopoxvirus or other poxvirus illnesses.
- In vitro, cidofovir is active against monkeypox; in vivo, it protects challenged animals when given prophylactically or early in the evolution of the disease.
  ○ In life-threatening cases, cidofovir may be administered but with hydration and probenecid because it is nephrotoxic.

Self-Management Strategies

- Contact and respiratory isolation precautions should be managed.
- Individuals who have been exposed should be monitored for fevers and symptoms for 21 days after the last known contact.[22]
- Vaccination with the smallpox vaccine is the mainstay for prevention of monkeypox (and other orthopoxvirus) infection. It should be given to anyone who has been exposed within 2 weeks (ideally 4 days of exposure), especially to veterinarians and veterinary technicians, who have had direct physical contact with an infected animal.[22]

Evaluation, Adjustment, Recurrence

Complications
Scarring, bacterial skin infections, respiratory and GI disorders, keratitis, septicemia, and encephalopathy.
Recurrence is rare.

EVALUATION AND WORKUP
Patient History

- Prodrome of fever, chills, diaphoresis, headache, backache, malaise, myalgia, and prostration
- Development of maculopapular rash begins on the trunk and spreads peripherally to involve the palms, soles, and mucous membranes. Pruritus may also be reported.

Physical Examination

- Clinical features are those similar to smallpox with the most obvious difference being pronounced submandibular, cervical, sublingual, and inguinal lymphadenopathy.
- Exanthem: nontender maculopapular rash with lesions usually 3 to 15 mm in diameter, begins on the trunk, palms, soles, and mucous membranes, evolves synchronously from vesicles → pustules → umbilication and then crusting in a 2- to 4-week period → resolution of rash → hypopigmentation followed by hyperpigmentation of the scarred lesions.[22]

Imaging and Additional Testing

Access to a virus diagnostic laboratory should permit detection of the virus with electron microscopy and molecular methods from viral cultures and skin biopsy. In some circumstances, distinguishing between monkeypox and tanapox may be important. Currently, an array of nucleic acid diagnostic techniques permits the speciation of the various orthopox viruses.

SMALLPOX

Smallpox is caused by infection of the upper respiratory mucosa by the orthopoxvirus variola. When prevalent, interhuman transmission generally occurs through the inhalation of large airborne respiratory droplets of infectious variola virus, but can also occur through contact with infected fomites or materials. Vaccination with smallpox vaccine was the primary method used to eradicate smallpox and is the key for prevention of orthopoxvirus infection.

Smallpox was initially subgrouped into 3 categories based on the extent of rash on the face and the body: ordinary confluent (no area of skin was visible between vesiculopustular rash lesions on the trunk or the face), semiconfluent (patches of normal skin were visible between lesions on the trunk), and discrete (patches of normal skin were visible between facial lesions). The World Health Organization (WHO) later classified smallpox into 4 main clinical types[1]:

1. Ordinary smallpox (90% of cases)
   a. Symptoms: Viremia, fever, prostration, and rash
2. Vaccine-modified smallpox (5% of cases)
   a. Mild prodrome with few skin lesions
3. Flat smallpox (5% of hospitalized cases)

a. Slowly developing lesions that appear flush with the edematous skin at the vesicular stage
b. Almost always fatal
c. Previous vaccination was protective against this form of the disease
4. Hemorrhagic smallpox (<1% of cases)
   a. Caused bleeding into the skin and the mucous membranes
   b. Previous vaccination was not protective against this form of the disease

A smallpox eradication program was developed in 1958 by WHO, and no cases of variola have occurred since 1977. In 1980, WHO declared the disease eradicated. The virus is kept at secure institutions in biosafety level 4 laboratories in the United States and Russia.[9]

MANAGEMENT STRATEGIES
Management Goals

Smallpox vaccine is currently recommended only for laboratory personnel who work with infectious orthopoxvirus, certain public health personnel, and certain members of the military.

Treatment Strategies

Currently, no antiviral drugs are licensed to treat orthopoxvirus or poxvirus illnesses.

Evaluation, Adjustment, Recurrence

- Mortality rate correlates directly with the rash burden.
- Mortality is more severe in children and pregnant women.
- Stockpiles of vaccine are available should smallpox recur.

EVALUATION AND WORKUP
Patient History

- Asymptomatic incubation period of 10 to 14 days followed by fever as high as 103°F.[9]
- Associated constitutional symptoms: Backache, headache, vomiting, extreme exhaustion, and fatigue.

Physical Examination

- Exanthem: Systemic centrifugal rash with lesions on the oral mucosa, face, and extremities. Lesions involve the palms and soles and are present in different clinical presentations ranging from macules and papules to vesicles (seen by day 4–5 of infection), pustules (seen by day 7), and encrusted and scabbed lesions.[9]

OTHER VIRAL ILLNESS WITH CUTANEOUS MANIFESTATIONS
Herpangina

- Virus: Coxsackie (most common cause), echovirus, HSV, and adenovirus[20]
- Transmitted by fecal-oral route or direct contact
- Predominantly affects children less than 10 years old[20]
- Typically seen in the summer or fall months
- Symptoms: fever and malaise → lymphadenopathy, sialorrhea, dysphagia → painful grayish-white papules → vesicles → ulcers (<5 mm in diameter) with a red rim on the soft palate, tonsils, uvula, and pharynx (**Fig. 36**)[20]

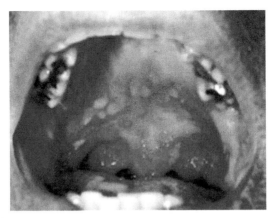

Fig. 36. Herpangina.

- ○ Absence of skin manifestations differentiates this from hand, foot, and mouth disease
- Diagnosis: Clinical diagnosis. Nasopharyngeal swab or serologic testing can be done but it is not warranted[10]
- Treatment: Supportive, analgesics, and adequate fluid intake. Usually resolves in 1 to 2 weeks. Cold drinks help to soothe the throat, while hot drinks should be avoided.

Infectious Mononucleosis

- Virus: EBV (most common cause) and cytomegalovirus (CMV)[10]
- Transmitted by direct contact with saliva or body fluids
- Symptoms: gradual onset of flulike symptoms → fever, pharyngitis, and tender lymphadenopathy (primarily the posterior cervical chain) ± splenomegaly, palatal petechiae, and in about 10%, a faint nonpruritic diffuse maculopapular rash appearing on the trunk and then disseminating to the extremities and face (see **Fig. 37**)

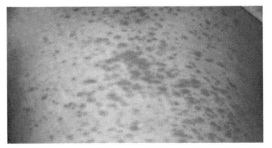

Fig. 37. Infectious mononucleosis.

- Patients with EBV can develop a pruritic nonallergic maculopapular rash on the extensor surfaces or pressure points 7 to 10 days after receiving ampicillin or amoxicillin[6]
- Diagnosis: Complete blood count with differential (CBC/D) with 50% lymphocytes (at least 10% atypical) and + monospot (heterophile antibody) test[1]

- Treatment: Supportive with analgesics, fluids, and rest. Avoid contact sports and other heavy physical activity that involve increased abdominal pressure (ie, rowing or weight-lifting) for at least 3 to 4 weeks and until splenomegaly has resolved as determined by a physician

Ebola

- Transmitted by direct contact with infected body fluids
- Symptoms: fever, flulike symptoms, headache, pharyngitis, and myalgia → emesis, diarrhea, maculopapular rash ± petechiae, purpura, ecchymosis, or hematomas, and decreased liver and renal function → internal and external bleeding (5–7 days after symptoms start)[1]
- Diagnosis: Laboratory tests: ↓ platelet, ↑ liver function tests, and signs associated with disseminated intravascular coagulation (↑ prothrombin time, partial thromboplastin time, and bleeding time). Definitive diagnosis with PCR[1]
- Strict infection control measures should be implemented, such as barrier isolation and wearing protective equipment.
- High mortality rate. Death usually occurs 6 to 16 days after initial symptoms due to hypotension from fluid loss.
- Recovery begins 1 to 2 weeks after first symptoms and provides immunity.[1]

Chikungunya Fever

- Virus: Chikungunya virus (Togaviridae family)[23]
- Transmitted by mosquito (not contagious) in tropical areas
- Symptoms: acute onset of fever, flulike symptoms, headache, severe debilitating arthralgia (beginning in the small joints and then the larger joints), and slightly raised maculopapular rash over the trunk, limb and face (**Fig. 38**)

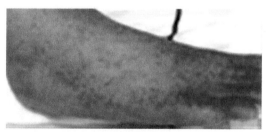

Fig. 38. Chikungunya fever.

- Diagnosis: ELISA or PCR.[23]
- Treatment: Supportive with optimal analgesics, fluids, and rest. Symptoms usually resolve within 1 week, but arthralgia may persist for months.[23]

Dengue Fever

- Virus: Dengue virus (5 subtypes of virus)
- Transmitted by mosquito bite (not contagious), primarily in tropical and subtropical areas[6]
- Symptoms: Acute-onset high fever, flulike symptoms, frontal headache, arthralgia, and rash (macular rash originating on the trunk → extremities and face). Rash is often referred to as "island of white in a sea of red."[6]
- Diagnosis: ELISA or PCR

Viral Hemorrhagic Fever

- Caused by 4 distinct RNA virus families: Arenavirus (Lassa, Argentine, Bolivian, Brazilian, and Venezuelan hemorrhagic fever), filovirus (Ebola and Marburg virus), bunyavirus (Hantavirus), and flavivirus (yellow and dengue fever)[6]
- Transmitted by aerosol or direct contact
- Multiple organs are affected. Specific signs and symptoms vary based on viral cause, but generally, patients have high fever, malaise, fatigue, and a maculopapular/petechial rash → bleeding and hemorrhage.[6]
- Treatment: supportive with pain relievers, fluids, and rest

Table 29 examines viral illnesses with rare cutaneous manifestations.

Table 29	
Viral illness with rare cutaneous manifestations	
Viral Illness	**Skin Manifestation**
Influenza	May sometimes present with a pinkish petechial rash that may become confluent sparing the face, palms, and soles
Alphavirus	Mosquito-transmitted viruses that cause multiple erythematous small papules
Herpes B virus	It is extremely rare in humans and result from a monkey bite or scratch; small vesicular lesions at the site of exposure; can cause severe brain damage
Boston exanthem disease	Caused by Echovirus 16; fever with subsequent development of pink maculopapular rash seen on the face, trunk, and occasionally on the extremities
Echovirus nonspecific exanthem	Varies echoviruses (2, 6, 9, 11, 19, and 25) can cause rubelliform, morbilliform, petechial, vesicular, or punctate macular eruptions
Eruptive pseudoangiomatosis	Caused by echovirus 25 and 32, CMV, EBV, and coxsackie virus. Small (2–4 mm) blanchable, red papules resembling cherry angiomas on the face, trunk, and limbs. There are usually ≤10 lesions and they resolve spontaneously in 10 d
Lipschutz ulcer	Rare. Painful genital ulcers, fever, and lymphadenopathy in young women; not a STD; associated with CMV and EBV
Rare poxvirus lesions	Rare zoonotic lesions include cowpox, pseudocowpox ("milker's nodule"), sealpox, tanapox, and yabapox. Cowpox causes a localized pustular exanthema, whereas other infections cause a localized nodular lesion that resolves within weeks to months

Vaccination

Tables 30 and **31** describe attenuated live vaccines and recombinant vaccines.

- Contraindications for live attenuated vaccines:
  o Pregnancy: if unimmunized, patient must wait until after delivery before being vaccinated.
- Immunodeficiency, including malignancy, receiving chemotherapy, immunosuppressive or biological medications, HIV (in certain cases), and congenital immunodeficiency. Women should avoid becoming pregnant within 3 months of vaccination (and 1 month for varicella).[5]

Table 30
Attenuated live vaccines

Vaccine	Recommendations
Influenza (nasal)	Individuals 2–49 y old; administered yearly[24]
Measles, mumps, rubella	• All children >1 y old: 1st dose at 12–15 mo, 2nd dose 4–6 y old or 28 d after 1st dose[24] • Postpubertal women, teachers, child care employees, and health care workers at increased risk; also can be given to AIDS patients • Recommended for people born after 1957, with immunization unknown, and with serologic test that does not indicate immunity • Do not give if received immunoglobulins or blood products 2 wk before or 3 mo after vaccination[24]
Smallpox	• Prevention for monkeypox and other orthopoxvirus infections ○ Monkeypox: Recommended for anyone who has been exposed within 2 wk (ideally 4 d of exposure), especially to veterinarians and veterinary technicians who have had direct physical contact with an infected animal[22] ○ Smallpox: Recommended only for laboratory personnel who work with infectious orthopoxvirus, certain public health personnel, and certain members of the military
Varicella	• Children <13 y old: 1st dose at 12–15 mo of age, 2nd dose at age 4–6 y • >13 y olds who have not had chickenpox or received vaccine should be fully vaccinated with 2 doses at least 28 d apart • Immunocompetent, >60-year-old individuals who are VZV seronegative • Adults who are at increased risk (such as day care and health care employees) • HIV patients with CD-4 count >350, 2 doses should be administered 3 mo apart
Yellow fever	9 mo of age and older in areas with high prevalence
Zoster	Immunocompetent adults ≥ age 60 regardless of previous episode of herpes zoster

Table 31
Recombinant vaccine

Vaccine	Recommendations
Influenza (IM, intradermal)	6 mo of age or older; administered yearly
HBV	• Children: 1st dose at birth, 2nd dose 1–2 mo old, 3rd dose 6–18 mo old • Unvaccinated adults at increased risk, include homosexual men, intravenous drug abuse, people with chronic liver or kidney disease, <60 y old with diabetes, health care worker, HIV positive
HPV	3 vaccines exist (either one can be given); decreases the risk cf genital warts and cervical, vaginal, vulvar, and anal cancer. All 3 types are given as 3 doses. Second dose 1 mo after the 1st dose and 3rd dose given 6 mo after the initial dose HPV 4 (Gardasil): Quadrivalent (types 6, 11, 16, 18) for males and females 9–26 y old HPV 2 (Cervarix): Bivalent (types 16, 18) for females 10–26 y old Gardasil 9: Recombinant 9-valent (6, 11, 16, 18, 31, 33, 45, 52, and 58) for females 9–26 y old and males 9–15 y old

SUMMARY

Diagnosis of a viral skin infection is based on a conglomeration of key components. Knowledge of pathognomonic features and pattern recognition are pivotal in differentiating the likely pathogen, predicting the course, and deciding if and to what extent treatment is warranted. Although most viral skin infections have an archetypal set of features, some have diverged from the classic description, such as HSV. Diagnosis is often confirmed by serology or nucleic acid testing and rarely by vial culture. In general, viral exanthems are self-limiting and treatment is supportive, with only a few having life-long sequelae.

REFERENCES

1. Dietrich A, Dye LR, Hessen MT, et al. First consult. Philadelphia: Elsevier; 2015. Last updated March 11, 2015. Web. Accessed January 2, 2015.
2. Romano M, Mailhot J, Wiss K. Viral exanthems: rubella, roseola, rubeola, enteroviruses. In: Romano M, editor. Treatment of skin disease: comprehensive therapeutic strategies. Philadelphia: Elsevier; 2013. p. 784–7.
3. Bello S, Meremikwu MM, Ejemot-Nwadiaro RI, et al. Routine vitamin A supplementation for the prevention of blindness due to measles infection in children. Cochrane Database Syst Rev 2011;(4):CD007719.
4. Kliegman RM, Nelson WE. Nelson textbook of pediatrics. Philadelphia: Elsevier Saunders; 2011.
5. Habif TP. Clinical dermatology: a color guide to diagnosis and therapy. 5th edition. Philadelphia: Elsevier; 2010.
6. Goldman L, Schafer AI, Cecil RL. Goldman's Cecil medicine. Philadelphia: Elsevier Saunders; 2012.
7. Jordan JA. Clinical manifestations and diagnosis of human parvovirus B19 infection. Uptodate; 2014.
8. Tremblay C, Brady MT. Roseola infantum (exanthem subitum). Uptodate; 2014.
9. DermNet NZ. Ed. Amanda Oakley M.D. N.p., 1996. Web. Nov.-Dec. 2014. http://www.dermnetnz.org/.
10. Ferri FF. 2015 Ferri's clinical advisor: 5 books in 1. Philadelphia: Elsevier; 2014.
11. Albrecht MA. Epidemiology, clinical manifestations, and diagnosis of genital herpes simplex virus infection. Uptodate; 2014.
12. Kimberlin DW, Rouse DJ. Genital herpes. N Engl J Med 2004;350(19):1970–7.
13. Centers for Disease Control and Prevention. Sexually transmitted diseases. Atlanta (GA): Centers for Disease Control and Prevention; 2013.
14. Murahwa AT, Muchemwa FC, Duri K, et al. Presence of Betapapillomavirus in Kaposi sarcoma lesions. J Med Virol 2014;86(9):1556–9.
15. Díaz-Ley B, Grillo E, Ríos-Buceta L, et al. Classic Kaposi's sarcoma treated with topical rapamycin. Dermatol Ther 2015;28(1):40–3.
16. Palefsky JM. Epidemiology of human papillomavirus infections. Uptodate; 2014.
17. Carusi DA. Epidemiology of human papillomavirus infections. Uptodate; 2014.
18. Breen E, Bleday R. Condylomata acuminata (anogenital warts) in adults. Uptodate; 2014.
19. Castle PE, Cox TJ, Palefsky JM. Recommendations for the use of human papillomavirus vaccines. Uptodate; 2014.
20. Romero JR. Hand, foot, and mouth disease and herpangina: an overview. Uptodate; 2014.
21. Isaacs SN. Molluscum contagiosum. Uptodate; 2014.
22. Isaacs SN. Monkeypox. Uptodate; 2014.

23. Wilson ME, Baron EL. Chikungunya fever. Uptodate; 2014.
24. McLean HQ, Fiebelkorn AP, Temte JL, et al. Prevention of measles, rubella, congenital rubella syndrome, and mumps, 2013: summary recommendations of the Advisory Committee on Immunization Practices (ACIP). MMWR Recomm Rep 2013;62:1–34.

Evaluation and Management of the Hair Loss Patient in the Primary Care Setting

Isabella Ahanogbe, MD[a], Alde Carlo P. Gavino, MD[b],*

KEYWORDS

- Dermatology • Systemic disease • Skin findings • Rheumatologic conditions
- Gastrointestinal conditions

KEY POINTS

- Alopecias are broadly classified as noncicatricial and cicatricial, the main difference being that cicatricial alopecias destroy and lead to the permanent loss of hair follicles.
- Although usually reversible, if they run a protracted course and are left untreated, noncicatricial alopecias may also eventuate into permanent hair loss.
- The evaluation of a hair loss patient should include a comprehensive clinical history and physical examination; appropriate laboratory testing; and if indicated, a scalp biopsy.
- Treatment methods vary depending on the type of alopecia, and include watchful waiting, topical and systemic formulations, surgery, and treatment of any underlying or associated conditions.
- Early diagnosis and the timely institution of appropriate treatment are extremely helpful and comforting to those affected by this disease.

INTRODUCTION

Alopecia (hair loss) is a common presenting problem in the primary care setting and is a source of great emotional angst for most patients. It affects men and women of all ages and can affect all hair-bearing areas of the body. Alopecia can be a primary process, or can be a manifestation of an underlying medical condition. Hair loss is classified as noncicatricial (nonscarring) or cicatricial, the main difference being that cicatricial alopecias lead to destruction, and usually permanent loss, of hair follicles. Noncicatricial alopecias include male and female androgenetic alopecia (male and female pattern hair loss), alopecia areata, telogen effluvium, tinea capitis, traction

[a] Manning Regional Health Care Center, Manning, IA 51455, USA; [b] Department of Dermatology, Dell Medical School, The University of Texas at Austin, 601 East 15th Street, Austin, TX 78701, USA
* Corresponding author.
E-mail address: cgavino.md@gmail.com

Prim Care Clin Office Pract 42 (2015) 569–589
http://dx.doi.org/10.1016/j.pop.2015.07.005
0095-4543/15/$ – see front matter © 2015 Elsevier Inc. All rights reserved.

alopecia, and trichotillomania. Although alopecias can usually be diagnosed with a good clinical history and physical examination, laboratory examinations are often used to aid in the diagnosis, and to determine if there is an underlying condition causing or contributing to the hair loss. When the diagnosis is not clear on clinical grounds, a scalp biopsy is a powerful tool that not only can clinch the diagnosis, but can also provide valuable prognostic information. Although some forms of alopecia resolve spontaneously with watchful waiting, topical and systemic therapies are available for the treatment of others.

The lifespan of human hair follicles is spent asynchronously cycling through a period of growth (anagen), a transitional period (catagen), and a period of rest (telogen) (**Fig. 1**). Scalp hair follicles spend most of their time in anagen, which lasts approximately 2 to 6 years.[1,2] At any given time, less that 1% of hair follicles are transitioning from growth to rest in the catagen period, which lasts about 3 weeks on the scalp.[1,2] The resting phase lasts about 2 to 3 months at the end of which exogen, the shedding of hair, occurs. The duration of each period varies with the location and kind of hair. On average, humans shed 50 to 150 hairs per day.[3]

CLASSIFICATION OF ALOPECIAS

Alopecias can be classified into two major categories: noncicatricial alopecias and cicatricial alopecias. Noncicatricial alopecias (**Table 1**) are a result of a process that affects the growth cycle without destroying the hair follicle. Noncicatricial alopecias include male and female pattern alopecia, alopecia areata, telogen effluvium, tinea capitis, traction alopecia, and trichotillomania. Cicatricial alopecias destroy the hair follicles and cause irreversible damage and permanent hair loss. Of note, noncicatricial alopecias may run a protracted course, and if left untreated, may lead to permanent hair loss.

Noncicatricial Alopecias

Androgenetic/pattern alopecia
Androgenetic alopecia, also known as pattern hair loss, is mainly caused by genetic influences that can be traced through family lines. In some women, the cause may

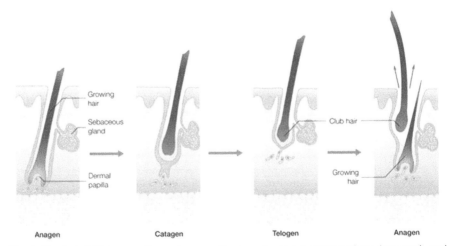

Fig. 1. The hair follicle goes through a growth phase (anagen), resting phase (catagen), and shedding phase (telogen). (*From* James WD, Berger T, Elston DMD. Andrews' diseases of the skin. 11th edition. Philadelphia: Saunders; 2011; with permission.)

Table 1
Noncicatricial alopecias

	Etiologies	Clinical Examination	Treatment
Focal alopecia			
Alopecia areata	Autoimmune	Smooth hairless patches; occasionally total scalp or body hair loss	Spontaneous remission; intralesional or topical steroids; immunotherapy
Alopecia syphilitica	Syphilis	"Moth eaten" appearance of patchy hair loss	2.4 million units of benzathine penicillin G (in patients without immunocompromise)[4]
Pressure induced (postoperative alopecia)	Extended pressure to scalp (ie, during anesthesia for long surgeries)[5]	Noncicatricial or cicatricial hair loss to contact area	Spontaneous resolution, although it may be permanent
Temporal triangular alopecia	Congenital	Unilateral or bilateral triangular or oval patch of alopecia temporally[6]	Hair transplantation[7]
Traction alopecia	Extended traction on hair follicles, generally caused by braids or tight ponytails	Hair loss to frontal and/or temporal hair lines	Avoidance of traction; cicatricial alopecia may occur
Patterned alopecia			
Male pattern hair loss	Genetic factors and action of androgen	Temporal, anterior, mid-scalp, and/or vertex scalp affected	Finasteride, dutasteride, minoxidil, surgery
Female pattern hair loss	Not fully clear, although hormonal and genetic predisposition contribute	Diffuse thinning with preservation of frontal hairline; "Christmas tree" pattern of thinning around central part	Finasteride, dutasteride, minoxidil, surgery
Trichotillomania	Impulse control disorder leading one to pull out hairs to achieve relief of tension	Irregular patches on scalp with hairs having varying lengths	Counseling; multidisciplinary approach; some medications with limited evidence
Diffuse alopecia			
Anagen effluvium	Disruption of anagen (chemotherapy, radiation)	Varying degree of thinning without scarring, erythema, or scaling	Withdrawal of inciting agent; minoxidil

(continued on next page)

Table 1
(*continued*)

	Etiologies	Clinical Examination	Treatment
Loose anagen hair syndrome	Sporadic; genetic factors (autosomal dominant)	Short, slowly growing hairs, easily pulled out, usually in blonde-haired females 2–5 y old	Observation; minoxidil[8]
Telogen effluvium	Major physical or psychological stressors, childbirth, medications, or metals	Increased hair loss perceived especially with washing or brushing[9]	Observation

Data from Refs.[4–8]

be hyperandrogenism.[10] The key finding in this disease is miniaturization of hair folli-cles. The clinical presentation in most women is that of diffuse thinning over the top of the scalp with preservation of the frontal hairline, creating a "Christmas tree" pattern of hair loss (**Figs. 2** and **3**). Female pattern alopecia typically does not progress to com-plete hair loss. In men, hair loss is progressive, and most commonly affects the vertex and temporal regions (**Figs. 4** and **5**).[11] Women with underlying hyperandrogenism may present with other signs or symptoms including abnormal menses, infertility, hir-sutism, or severe acne.[12] Androgenetic alopecia, for the most part, may be reliably diagnosed through clinical history and physical examination alone. Laboratory exam-inations, such as serum levels of testosterone and dehydroepiandrosterone sulfate, are helpful in determining the patient's androgen status. A skin biopsy is appropriate when the diagnosis is uncertain, and is usually done to differentiate pattern alopecia from telogen effluvium, because they may mimic each other, especially in women. Treatment is aimed primarily at reversing the miniaturization of hair follicles. In men and women, pattern alopecia can be devastating and may cause depression, low self-esteem, or dissatisfaction with body appearance.[13]

Alopecia areata

Alopecia areata is an autoimmune disorder that presents most commonly as acute patchy hair loss on the scalp (**Fig. 6**). Other types include alopecia areata totalis

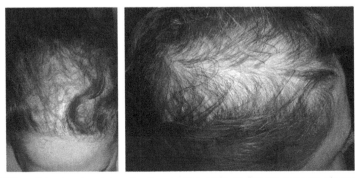

Fig. 2. Diffuse thinning involving the top of the scalp in female pattern alopecia. (*From* Restrepo R, Caonje JE. Diseases of the hair. In: Calonje JE, Brenn T, Lazar AJ, et al., editors. McKee's pathology of the skin. 4th edition. Philadelphia: Saunders; 2011; with permission.)

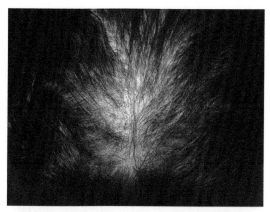

Fig. 3. Preservation of the frontal hair line in female pattern alopecia, creating the "Christmas tree" pattern. (*From* Restrepo R, Caonje JE. Diseases of the hair. In: Calonje JE, Brenn T, Lazar AJ, et al., editors. McKee's pathology of the skin. 4th edition. Philadelphia: Saunders; 2011; with permission.)

(loss of all scalp hair, **Fig. 7**) and alopecia areata universalis (loss of all scalp and body hair). The disease affects children and adults. Patients may have a singular episode or may experience several periods of remission and recurrence over many years. The diagnosis can usually be made on clinical grounds alone, but a scalp biopsy may be helpful in challenging cases. Pitting or trachyonychia (**Fig. 8**) are associated nail findings that may be seen in some patients, and may be helpful clues to the diagnosis.[14,15] For most patients, the disease resolves spontaneously within a year.[16] Treatment is aimed at stopping the inflammation attacking the hair follicles. Recently, several genetic variations associated with the development of alopecia areata have been identified, paving the way for better understanding of the pathophysiology of this disease, and for the development of targeted therapies.

Telogen effluvium

Telogen effluvium is another common form of noncicatricial alopecia (**Fig. 9**). It is caused by excessive shedding of telogen hairs and can affect men and women of any age. Inciting events include serious illnesses, major surgeries, childbirth, rapid weight loss, drug exposure (**Box 1**), or emotional stress. The trigger occurs up to

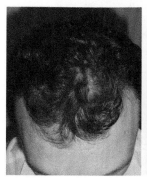
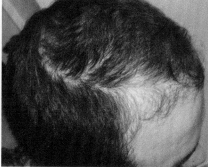

Fig. 4. Recession and thinning of the temporal scalp in male pattern alopecia. (*From* Restrepo R, Caonje JE. Diseases of the hair. In: Calonje JE, Brenn T, Lazar AJ, et al., editors. McKee's pathology of the skin. 4th edition. Philadelphia: Saunders; 2011; with permission.)

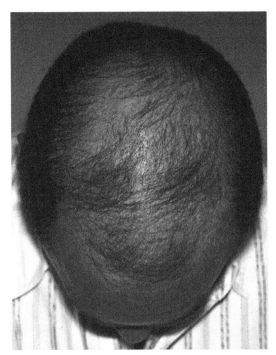

Fig. 5. Diffuse thinning involving the temporal scalp and vertex in advanced male pattern alopecia. (*From* James WD, Berger T, Elston DMD. Andrews' diseases of the skin. 11th edition. Philadelphia: Saunders; 2011; with permission.)

3 months before hair loss ensues.[17,18] The disease usually resolves spontaneously with time and with removal of the inciting event.[17,19]

Tinea capitis
Tinea capitis is a fungal infection of the scalp caused by dermatophytes. It usually occurs in younger children of African American or Afro-Caribbean descent,[20] and is

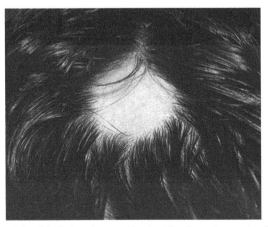

Fig. 6. A circular patch of hair loss in a patient with alopecia areata. (*From* Restrepo R, Caonje JE. Diseases of the hair. In: Calonje JE, Brenn T, Lazar AJ, et al., editors. McKee's pathology of the skin. 4th edition. Philadelphia: Saunders; 2011; with permission.)

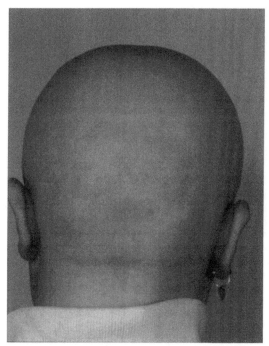

Fig. 7. Loss of all hairs on the scalp in a patient with alopecia areata totalis. (*From* Restrepo R, Caonje JE. Diseases of the hair. In: Calonje JE, Brenn T, Lazar AJ, et al., editors. McKee's pathology of the skin. 4th edition. Philadelphia: Saunders; 2011; with permission.)

spread by contact with fallen infected hairs and pets. It presents as discrete patches of alopecia studded with black dots ("black dot sign") that result from increased fragility of hairs and their subsequent breakage at the point where they emerge from the scalp (**Fig. 10**). Patients may also present with diffuse scaly plaques that may be mistaken for psoriasis or seborrheic dermatitis. Other patients may develop a kerion (**Fig. 11**), a markedly inflamed abscess that may lead to scarring.[19] Posterior cervical lymphadenopathy usually accompanies tinea capitis. Diagnosis of tinea capitis can be made by

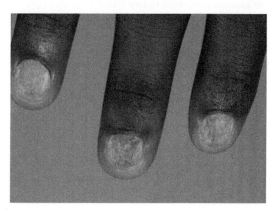

Fig. 8. Trachyonychia in a patient with alopecia areata. (*From* Sperling LC, Sinclair RD, Shabrawi-Caelen LE. Alopecias. In: Bolognia JL, Jorizzo JL, Schaffer JV, editors. Dermatology. 3rd edition. Philadelphia: Saunders; 2012; with permission.)

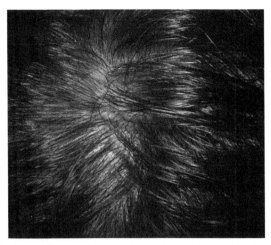

Fig. 9. Diffuse thinning without scale or erythema in a patient with telogen effluvium. The clinical appearance may be difficult to distinguish from pattern alopecia, especially in women. (*From* Restrepo R, Caonje JE. Diseases of the hair. In: Calonje JE, Brenn T, Lazar AJ, et al., editors. McKee's pathology of the skin. 4th edition. Philadelphia: Saunders; 2011; with permission.)

examination of hairs and scales under the microscope, by culture, or by doing a skin biopsy (reveals periodic acid Schiff–positive fungi). Wood lamp examination can also be used, although *Trichophyton tonsurans*, the most common causative organism in the United States, is not fluorescent.

Traction alopecia

Traction alopecia is another common form of hair loss usually seen in African American females who wear tight braids and tight ponytails. The disease results from constant and repetitive pulling of hairs, displacing them from their follicles, which then get damaged. Patients present with a band of thinning along the frontal and temporal scalp (**Fig. 12**). Once recognized, patients must be advised to stop hair practices

---

Box 1
Medications that may cause or contribute to hair loss

Anticoagulants (eg, warfarin, heparin)

Oral contraceptives

β-Blockers (eg, propranolol)

Anabolic steroids

Isotretinoin

Ketoconazole

Anticonvulsants (eg, valproic acid)

Antithyroid agents

Chemotherapy agents

Lithium

Colchicine

Captopril

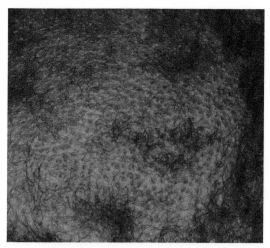

Fig. 10. Black dots on a patch of alopecia in a patient with tinea capitis. (*From* Elewski BE, Hughey LC, Sobera JO, et al. Fungal diseases. In: Bolognia JL, Jorizzo JL, Schaffer JV, editors. Dermatology. 3rd edition. Philadelphia: Saunders; 2012; with permission.)

that involve pulling their hairs. Although initially noncicatricial, traction alopecia over time may lead to permanent loss of hairs.[19]

Trichotillomania

Trichotillomania involves the persistent plucking of one's own hairs. It is an impulse control disorder that is the most common cause of childhood alopecia.[19,21,22] It occurs equally in men and women, with a typical age of onset of 8 years in boys and 12 years in girls. Patients present with patches of alopecia, with hairs often having varying

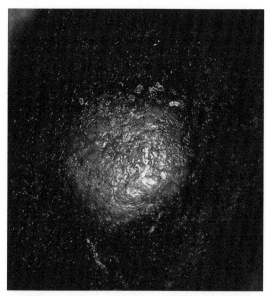

Fig. 11. Kerion formation in a patient with tinea capitis. (*From* Elewski BE, Hughey LC, Sobera JO, et al. Fungal diseases. In: Bolognia JL, Jorizzo JL, Schaffer JV, editors. Dermatology. 3rd edition. Philadelphia: Saunders; 2012; with permission.)

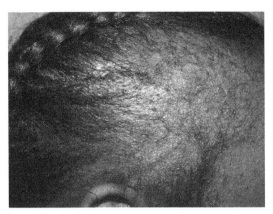

Fig. 12. Thinning on the temporal scalp in a patient with traction alopecia. Note how tightly the patient's hair is pulled back. Over time, if traction continues, hair loss becomes permanent. (*From* Sperling LC, Sinclair RD, Shabrawi-Caelen LE. Alopecias. In: Bolognia JL, Jorizzo JL, Schaffer JV, editors. Dermatology. 3rd edition. Philadelphia: Saunders; 2012; with permission.)

lengths (**Fig. 13**). The disease is characterized by (1) recurrent pulling out of one's hair, resulting in hair loss; (2) repeated attempts to decrease or stop hair pulling; (3) the hair pulling causes clinically significant distress or impairment in social, occupational, or other important areas of functioning; (4) the hair pulling or hair loss is not attributable to another medical condition; and (5) the hair pulling is not better explained by the symptoms of another mental disorder. Patients describe increased emotional tension before pulling out hair, and relief after the hair is pulled out. Patients often do not acknowledge that they are pulling their hair, and family members may not witness them doing so. Some patients engage in trichophagia (eating of hair), and may develop

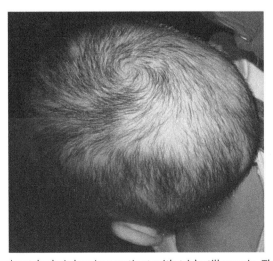

Fig. 13. Diffuse and patchy hair loss in a patient with trichotillomania. The clinical appearance may be difficult to distinguish from alopecia areata. A careful clinical history and physical examination, sometimes aided by a scalp biopsy, and a high index of suspicion are needed to clinch the diagnosis. (*From* Restrepo R, Caonje JE. Diseases of the hair. In: Calonje JE, Brenn T, Lazar AJ, et al., editors. McKee's pathology of the skin. 4th edition. Philadelphia: Saunders; 2011; with permission.)

complications, such as formation of trichobezoars, which are hairs stuck in the stomach or intestines; skin infections; and psychological problems, such as low self-esteem.[19,23] Cognitive behavioral therapy, specifically habit reversal therapy, may improve symptom severity and may be more effective than pharmacotherapy. Medications that may decrease symptom severity include olanzapine, N-acetylcysteine, and clomipramine. A multidisciplinary approach to management that involves a psychologist and/or psychiatrist, the primary care physician, the dermatologist, and family members is most ideal.

Cicatricial Alopecias

Cicatricial alopecias are divided into two groups: primary and secondary.[24] Primary cicatricial alopecias are inflammatory disorders further classified as lymphocytic, neutrophilic, or mixed (**Box 2**).[25,26] This subclassification is based on the predominant inflammatory cell type involved in the pathogenesis of the disease. Secondary cicatricial alopecia is characterized by permanent destruction of hair follicles because of an infectious, inflammatory, traumatic, or neoplastic (usually metastatic) process.[27] Cicatricial alopecia can affect men and women of all ages. The clinical presentation depends on the specific disease, and may include hyperpigmentation or hypopigmentation, itching, pain, erythema, plaques, papules, pustules, nodules, and scarring (**Figs. 14–18**).[25,26] Other hair-bearing areas of the body may be affected, so a full body examination is an important part of the evaluation of the patient. Once a cicatricial process is suspected, a scalp biopsy should be performed to establish the diagnosis. The biopsy is best done at sites of active disease where characteristic histologic changes would be present. Areas of complete balding should be avoided, because a biopsy from such area would just yield nonspecific fibrosis.[28] Treatment modalities for cicatricial alopecias include topical/intralesional/systemic steroids, antibiotics, antimalarial drugs, nonsteroidal anti-inflammatory medications, and androgen inhibitors.

Box 2
Cicatricial alopecias

Lymphocytic primary cicatricial alopecias

Discoid lupus erythematous

Frontal fibrosing alopecia

Lichen planopilaris

Pseudopelade

Alopecia mucinosa

Keratosis follicularis spinulosa decalvans

Central centrifugal cicatricial alopecia

Neutrophilic primary cicatricial alopecias

Dissecting cellulitis

Folliculitis decalvans

Mixed primary cicatricial alopecias

Acne keloidalis nuchae

Acne necrotica

Erosive pustular dermatosis of the scalp

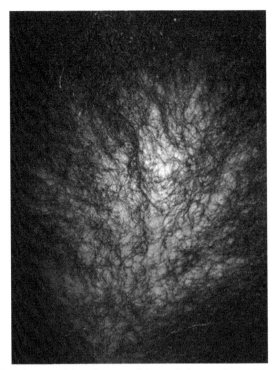

Fig. 14. Scarring hair loss involving the top of the scalp in a patient with central centrifugal cicatricial alopecia. (*From* Sperling LC, Sinclair RD, Shabrawi-Caelen LE. Alopecias. In: Bolognia JL, Jorizzo JL, Schaffer JV, editors. Dermatology. 3rd edition. Philadelphia: Saunders; 2012; with permission.)

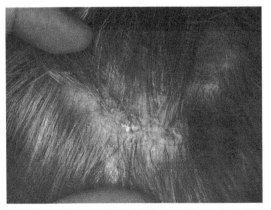

Fig. 15. Perifollicular erythema in a patient with lichen planopilaris. (*From* Sperling LC, Sinclair RD, Shabrawi-Caelen LE. Alopecias. In: Bolognia JL, Jorizzo JL, Schaffer JV, editors. Dermatology. 3rd edition. Philadelphia: Saunders; 2012; with permission.)

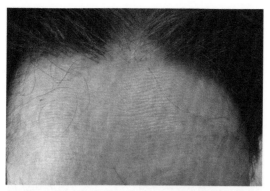

Fig. 16. Bandlike recession of the frontal hair line and perifollicular erythema in a patient with frontal fibrosing alopecia, a variant of lichen planopilaris. (*From* Bolognia JL, Jorizzo JL, Schaffer JV. Dermatology. 3rd edition. Philadelphia: Saunders; 2012; with permission.)

APPROACH TO THE PATIENT WITH ALOPECIA
Diagnosis

The diagnosis of alopecia may be made with the clinical history and physical examination alone. However, there are instances, especially when dealing with cicatricial alopecias, when a biopsy is necessary. Laboratory studies are also often helpful.

Clinical history

- History of present illness: An account of the date of onset, duration, acuity or chronicity, previous similar occurrences, and possible inciting events of the hair loss can provide a great deal of information to aid in the diagnosis of alopecia. A self-description of changes perceived (eg, asking the patient how much reduction there has been in the circumference of their ponytail) conveys the extent of hair loss, because alopecia is not appreciated by another person until approximately 30% of the baseline hair volume has been lost.[29] Patients should be asked about their hair styling and hair care practices.

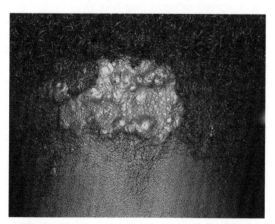

Fig. 17. Keloidal scarring on the occipital scalp in a patient with acne keloidalis nuchae. (*From* McMichael A, Curtis AR, Guzman-Sanchez D. Folliculitis and other follicular disorders. In: Bolognia JL, Jorizzo JL, Schaffer JV, editors. Dermatology. 3rd edition. Philadelphia: Saunders; 2012; with permission.)

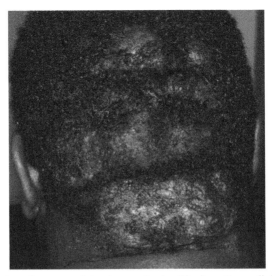

Fig. 18. Inflammatory, boggy nodules in a patient with dissecting cellulitis. (*From* McMichael A, Curtis AR, Guzman-Sanchez D. Folliculitis and other follicular disorders. In: Bolognia JL, Jorizzo JL, Schaffer JV, editors. Dermatology. 3rd edition. Philadelphia: Saunders; 2012; with permission.)

- Review of systems: A comprehensive review of systems, including psychiatric and neurologic symptoms, should be performed when evaluating a patient with alopecia. Fever or chills could support an underlying systemic cause. Weight loss or gain, nail changes, hirsutism, abnormal menses, or changes in the quality of voice may reveal an underlying endocrine disorder. Rashes, gastrointestinal symptoms, or joint and muscle aches could be caused by an underlying autoimmune disorder.
- Medications: Past and current medications should be reviewed to identify those that may cause or worsen alopecia (see **Box 1**).
- Past medical history: One should ask about recent or chronic medical illnesses (eg, iron deficiency anemia or thyroid disease), major surgery, rapid weight loss, dietary restrictions, recent childbirth, and miscarriage or abortion because these may cause telogen effluvium. Irregular menses, infertility, or hirsutism can point to a possible hormonal imbalance that is contributing to pattern alopecia. Alopecia areata may be present in the setting of other autoimmune disorders, such as diabetes, vitiligo, systemic lupus erythematosus, Hashimoto thyroiditis, and celiac disease.[14] Psychiatric conditions, such as anxiety, posttraumatic stress disorder, or psychosis, may trigger trichotillomania. Possible exposure to arsenic, mercury, or other toxins should also be elicited.
- Social history: Evaluate for recent stressors that may have caused telogen effluvium. Females involved in sports who wear their hair in tight ponytails for prolonged periods of time may present with traction alopecia. A sexual history could uncover syphilis as a possible cause of alopecia. Inquiries about a person's occupation are helpful in toxic chemical exposure or ingestion. Questions on dietary and exercise habits reveal any caloric or protein deficits. Smoking history and the amount of exposure to ultraviolet radiation are other factors that may have a role in the causation or worsening of alopecia.[10]

- Family history: The patient should be asked about family members with hair loss, especially in the setting of pattern alopecia. Other pertinent family history, particularly when evaluating a patient with alopecia areata, includes atopy, autoimmune disorders, and Down syndrome.[14]

Physical examination

The physical examination should be conducted under good lighting with the clinician comfortably visualizing the entire scalp. The examination of a person with alopecia of the scalp should include the nails, oral mucosa, and the rest of the body, with a focus on hair-bearing areas, such as the face, axillae, and groin.

The clinician should first determine whether the patient's hair loss is diffuse or focal. Diffuse hair loss should further be examined by parting hairs and noting the amount of space between partitions and comparing these areas with other sections of the scalp.[12] Attention should also be paid to any scales, pustules, or excoriations. The hair shafts should then be examined for length, shape, texture, and fragility.[10,12]

The pull test or traction test[30] is useful in the evaluation of diffuse hair loss and is suggestive of active hair shedding when six or more hairs are pulled out from a single area. It is performed by grasping 40 to 60 hairs at their base using the thumb, index, and middle fingers and applying gentle traction away from the scalp.[31,32] A positive test suggests telogen effluvium, anagen effluvium, or the advancing edge of alopecia areata, but a negative test does not necessarily exclude those diseases.[33] In addition, if the patient washed their scalp before the clinic visit, the pull test would be negative because the telogen hairs would have already been shed.

The wash test is another clinical tool used to evaluate diffuse alopecia. It is conducted by collecting hairs shed after washing the scalp. The patient is asked to not wash their scalp for 5 days before the test.[33] Shed hairs are then counted and separated into groups by length of 5 cm or longer, between 3 and 5 cm, and 3 cm or shorter. Those that are shorter than 3 cm are counted as telogen vellus hairs. A 10% or greater count of telogen vellus hairs suggests the diagnosis of pattern alopecia.[34]

Trichoscopy is a technique based on dermoscopy and videodermoscopy used to assess the scalp and hair under high magnification.[35] Special training to perform and master this skill is available and could be extremely valuable, especially to the clinician who sees a lot of hair loss patients. Trichoscopy can be helpful in evaluating the diameter of hair shafts; an increased number of miniaturized hairs supports the diagnosis of pattern alopecia.[30,36] It can help differentiate pattern alopecia from telogen effluvium in that the latter is characterized by the presence of empty follicles.[36] Characteristic trichoscopic features of alopecia areata include yellow dots, black dots, broken hairs, and exclamation mark hairs (**Fig. 19**). Trichotillomania may also have yellow and black dots on trichoscopy, and may thus be difficult to differentiate from alopecia areata. However, trichotillomania may have coiled hairs.[36,37] "Comma hairs," which appear as slightly curved, fractured hair shafts are seen in active lesions of tinea capitis.[38] Trichoscopy can also be helpful in the evaluation of cicatricial alopecias. For example, in patients with discoid lupus erythematous, trichoscopy can reveal diagnostic clues, such as follicular plugs, arborizing vessels, white patches, and blue-grey dots.[36,39]

The scalp biopsy

A scalp biopsy is an important tool in the evaluation and management of alopecias. It is indicated in all cases of cicatricial alopecia,[40] and is performed when the precise diagnosis of a noncicatricial alopecia is in question. A scalp biopsy not only helps in the diagnosis of hair loss, but can only provide invaluable prognostic information.

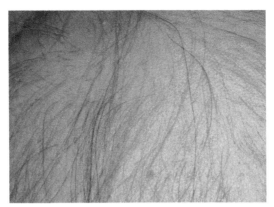

Fig. 19. "Exclamation mark" hairs in alopecia areata. (*From* Sperling LC, Sinclair RD, Shabrawi-Caelen LE. Alopecias. In: Bolognia JL, Jorizzo JL, Schaffer JV, editors. Dermatology. 3rd edition. Philadelphia: Saunders; 2012; with permission.)

The biopsy is performed by first injecting the site with 1% lidocaine containing epinephrine. It is recommended that the biopsy be performed 15 minutes later, because it takes that long for the vasoconstrictive effect of epinephrine to start working. This helps prevent excessive bleeding during the procedure. A 4-mm punch biopsy is the gold standard[15] and should be the only diameter used when obtaining a sample for the evaluation of alopecias.

The sample is then sent to the laboratory where it should be horizontally sectioned, allowing the pathologist to evaluate all the hair follicles at once (**Fig. 20**).[41,42] Only one biopsy is necessary for most alopecias. In the evaluation of pattern alopecia, however, two biopsies may be helpful. One biopsy is obtained from the top of the scalp, and the other is obtained from the occipital scalp. This allows the pathologist to compare the two sites, using the occipital scalp as the "normal" sample because pattern alopecia typically does not affect that area.

Evaluation of the scalp biopsy involves counting the total number of hair follicles, and the numbers of anagen, catagen/telogen, and vellus/miniaturized hairs.[43] The anagen to catagen/telogen and the terminal to vellus hair ratios are then calculated. The pathologist also notes the presence of inflammation and fibrosis. These pieces of information are then put together and a diagnosis is rendered.

Management

Laboratory work-up
Laboratory testing is not normally needed for the diagnosis of hair loss, although it can be used to support a particular diagnosis or to evaluate an associated or underlying condition. **Table 2** lists some of the laboratory tests that are helpful in the management of certain types of alopecia.

Treatment
First-line treatments for male pattern alopecia include minoxidil and finasteride. Finasteride may be more efficacious than minoxidil,[47] but they yield even better results when used together. Response to treatment varies from regrowth to slowing of additional hair loss, and should be assessed after 12 months of continued use. To maintain the results achieved from these medications, therapy must be continued indefinitely. In a small proportion of patients, finasteride may cause sexual dysfunction and a

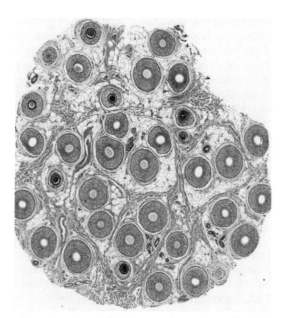

Fig. 20. A horizontally sectioned scalp biopsy. Note how this method allows visualization of all the hair follicles at once. (H&E). (*From* Sperling LC, Sinclair RD, Shabrawi-Caelen LE. Alopecias. In: Bolognia JL, Jorizzo JL, Schaffer JV, editors. Dermatology. 3rd edition. Philadelphia: Saunders; 2012; with permission.)

decline in prostate-specific antigen.[48] Hair transplantation is another treatment option, and has been refined over the years, resulting in better outcomes for patients.[49]

Topical minoxidil is first-line treatment of female pattern alopecia. The medication is available in 2% and 5% concentrations, and in solution and foam formulations. Scalp pruritus, flaking, and facial trichosis are potential side effects, and are reported more with use of the solution than the foam.[50] It is important to instruct the patient to apply

Table 2
Laboratory studies that may be helpful in the diagnosis and management of alopecias

Laboratory Studies	Conditions
Prolactin, FSH, LH, DHEA-S	FPA, hyperandrogenism
Iron studies[44]	FPA, alopecia areata, anemia
Nontreponemal and treponemal antigen tests (RPR, FTA-ABS, and VDRL)[45]	Alopecia syphilitica, telogen effluvium
Erythrocyte sedimentation rate, rheumatoid factor, autoantibody blood tests[45]	Systemic lupus erythematosus, autoimmune disorders
Specimen examination with potassium hydroxide under microscopy[20]	Tinea capitis
Thyroid function tests[14,15,46]	Alopecia areata, FPA
Vitamin D levels[15]	Alopecia areata, FPA

Abbreviations: DHEA-S, dehydroepiandrosterone-sulfate; FPA, female pattern alopecia; FSH, follicle-stimulating hormone; FTA-ABS, fluorescent treponemal antibody absorption; LH, luteinizing hormone; RPR, rapid plasma reagin.
Data from Refs.[14,15,20,44–46]

minoxidil to the scalp and not the hair. They should wash their hands thoroughly after applying the medication; alternatively, they can wear gloves. Minoxidil may induce hair growth in areas of body that it comes into contact with other than the scalp. It is also very important to inform the patient that increased hair shedding may occur during the first 2 to 8 weeks of treatment because minoxidil induces follicles to shed their hairs to allow for new growth; patients should be assured that this is a sign the medication is working.[50,51] Minoxidil should be used for at least a year to assess efficacy. Although women do not completely go bald with progression of pattern alopecia, minoxidil should be used indefinitely for continued results. Systemic treatment options include spironolactone, cyproterone acetate[52] (not available in the United States), and finasteride. Spironolactone may be administered at a maximum dose of 200 mg daily, titrated up from a starting dose of 50 mg per day. It should be continued for at least 6 months before assessing effectiveness.[30] Serum potassium levels and blood pressure should be monitored closely, and spironolactone should be avoided in pregnancy.[53] Hair transplantation is a good option for women who fail to show improvement with pharmacologic therapy.[54,55] Cosmetic aids, such as wigs, are of great use, and in the management of the female patient with pattern alopecia.

Most cases of alopecia areata resolve completely over a period of 6 to 12 months, even in the absence of treatment. Patients usually opt to treat the disease, however, given the physical, emotional, and social impact it has on them. Treatment options include intralesional triamcinolone acetonide at a dose of 5 to 10 mg/mL, administered every 4 to 6 weeks as multiple superficial injections throughout the alopecic patches. Another treatment option is the use of potent topical corticosteroids, applied twice a day to the affected areas.[56] Extensive or recalcitrant disease may be successfully treated with topical immunotherapy by a dermatologist.[45] Immunotherapy agents include diphenylcyclopropenone, squaric acid dibutyl ester, or dinitrochlorobenzene.

The treatment of tinea capitis requires systemic antifungals. Terbinafine is the first-line agent when treating tinea caused by *Trichophyton*. It can be given in children as young as 4 years old. Dosing is based on weight: 62.5 mg/day for 2 to 4 weeks for children 10 to 20 kg; 125 mg/day for 2 to 4 weeks for children 20 to 40 kg; and 250 mg/day for 2 to 4 weeks for adults and for children greater than 40 kg. Griseofulvin dosing is 10 to 25 mg/kg/day for 6 to 12 weeks depending on the formulation for children[57]; for adults it is 10 to 15 mg/kg/day with a maximum dose of 750 mg per day.[58] Itraconazole and fluconazole are other options for the treatment of tinea capitis.[57] Ketoconazole should not be used in the treatment of tinea capitis.[59]

When to refer to a dermatologist

Cicatricial alopecias are best evaluated by a dermatologist.[12] Prompt diagnosis and treatment are important in cicatricial alopecias because the hair follicles cannot be regenerated once they are permanently destroyed. Referral to a dermatologist may also be helpful in noncicatricial alopecias, especially when the diagnosis is challenging, or when conventional treatment modalities have failed to improve or resolve the disease.

SUMMARY

Alopecias represent a heterogeneous group of disorders with different etiologies, presentations, and treatment options. They are broadly classified as noncicatricial and cicatricial, the main difference being that cicatricial alopecias destroy and lead to the permanent loss of hair follicles. Although usually reversible, if they run a protracted course and are left untreated, noncicatricial alopecias may also eventuate into permanent hair loss. The evaluation of a hair loss patient should include a comprehensive clinical history and physical examination; appropriate laboratory testing; and if indicated, a scalp biopsy. Treatment methods vary depending on the type of alopecia, and include watchful waiting, topical and systemic formulations, surgery, and treatment of any underlying or associated conditions. Referral to a dermatologist is helpful in diagnostically challenging and difficult to treat cases. Alopecia can cause a great deal of emotional, mental, and social distress to patients. Early diagnosis and the timely institution of appropriate treatment are extremely helpful and comforting to those affected by this disease.

REFERENCES

1. Breitkopf T, Leung G, Yu M, et al. The basic science of hair biology: what are the causal mechanisms for the disordered hair follicle? Dermatol Clin 2013;31:1.
2. Price VH. Treatment of hair loss. N Engl J Med 1999;341:964.
3. Paus R, Cotsarelis G. The biology of hair follicles. N Engl J Med 1999;341:491.
4. Bi MY, Cohen PR, Robinson FW, et al. Alopecia syphilitica: report of a patient with secondary syphilis presenting as moth-eaten alopecia and a review of its common mimickers. Dermatol Online J 2009;15(10):6.
5. Wiles JC, Hansen RC. Postoperative (pressure) alopecia. J Am Acad Dermatol 1985;12:195.
6. Yamazaki M, Irisawa R, Tsuboi R. Temporal triangular alopecia and a review of 52 past cases. J Dermatol 2010;37:360.
7. Chung J, Sim JH, Gye J, et al. Successful hair transplantation for treatment of acquired temporal triangular alopecia. Dermatol Surg 2012;38:1404.
8. Cantatore-Francis JL, Orlow SJ. Practical guidelines for evaluation of loose anagen hair syndrome. Arch Dermatol 2009;145:1123–8.
9. de Berker D. Clinical relevance of hair microscopy in alopecia. Clin Exp Dermatol 2002;27:366–72.
10. Blume-Peytavi U, Blumeyer A, Tosti A, et al, European Consensus Group. S1 guideline for diagnostic evaluation in androgenetic alopecia in men, women and adolescents. Br J Dermatol 2011;164(1):5–15.
11. Van Zuuren EJ, Fedorowicz Z, Carter B, et al. Interventions for female pattern hair loss. Cochrane Database Syst Rev 2012;5:CD007628. Summary can be found in Br J Dermatol 2012;167(5):995–1010.
12. Mounsey AL, Reed SW. Diagnosing and treating hair loss. Am Fam Physician 2009;80(4):356–62.
13. Stough D, Stenn K, Haber R, et al. Psychological effect, pathophysiology, and management of androgenetic alopecia in men. Mayo Clin Proc 2005;80(10):1316–22. Commentary can be found in Mayo Clin Proc 2006;81(2):267.
14. Gilhar A, Etzioni A, Paus R. Alopecia areata. N Engl J Med 2012;366(16):1515–25. Commentary can be found in N Engl J Med 2012;367(3):279.
15. Gordon KA, Tosti A. Alopecia: evaluation and treatment. Clin Cosmet Investig Dermatol 2011;4:101–6.
16. Bertolino AP. Alopecia areata. A clinical overview. Postgrad Med 2000;107:81–5, 89–90.
17. Sperling LC, Mezebish DS. Hair diseases. Med Clin North Am 1998;82:1155–69.
18. Jackson EA. Hair disorders. Prim Care 2000;27:319–32.
19. Springer K, Brown M, Stulberg DL. Common hair loss disorders. Am Fam Physician 2003;68(1):93–102.
20. Andrews MD, Burns M. Common tinea infections in children. Am Fam Physician 2008;77(10):1415–20.

21. Christenson GA, Crow SJ. The characterization and treatment of trichotillomania. J Clin Psychiatry 1996;57(Suppl 8):42–7.
22. Messinger ML, Cheng TL. Trichotillomania. Pediatr Rev 1999;20:249–50.
23. Duke DC, Keeley ML, Geffken GR, et al. Trichotillomania: a current review. Clin Psychol Rev 2010;30(2):181–93.
24. Olsen EA, Bergfeld WF, Cotsarelis G, et al. Summary of North American Hair Research Society (NAHRS)-sponsored workshop on cicatricial alopecia, Duke University Medical Center, February 10 and 11, 2001. J Am Acad Dermatol 2003;48:103.
25. Otberg N, Shapiro J. Hair growth disorders. In: Goldsmith LA, Katz SI, Gilchrest BA, et al, editors. Fitzpatrick's dermatology in general medicine. 8th edition. New York: McGraw Hill; 2012.
26. Childs JM, Sperling LC. Histopathology of scarring and nonscarring hair loss. Dermatol Clin 2013;31:43.
27. Thakur BK, Verma S. Is hair transplantation always successful in secondary cicatricial alopecia? Int J Trichology 2015;7(1):43–4.
28. Ross EK, Tan E, Shapiro J. Update on primary cicatricial alopecias. J Am Acad Dermatol 2005;53:1.
29. Moghadam-Kia S, Franks AG Jr. Autoimmune disease and hair loss. Dermatol Clin 2013;31:75.
30. Camacho-Martinez FM. Hair loss in women. Semin Cutan Med Surg 2009;28:19–32.
31. Hillmann K, Blume-Peytavi U. Diagnosis of hair disorders. Semin Cutan Med Surg 2009;28(1):33–8.
32. Van Neste MD. Assessment of hair loss: clinical relevance of hair growth evaluation methods. Clin Exp Dermatol 2002;27:362–9.
33. Dhurat R, Saraogi P. Hair evaluation methods: merits and demerits. Int J Trichology 2009;1(2):108–19.
34. Rebora A, Guarrera M, Baldari M, et al. Distinguishing androgenetic alopecia from chronic telogen effluvium when associated in the same patient: a simple noninvasive method. Arch Dermatol 2005;141(10):1243–5.
35. Rakowska A. Trichoscopy (hair and scalp videodermoscopy) in the healthy female. Method standardization and norms for measurable parameters. J Dermatol Case Rep 2009;3(1):14–9.
36. Tosti A, Torres F. Dermoscopy in the diagnosis of hair and scalp disorders. Actas Dermosifiliogr 2009;100(Suppl 1):114–9.
37. Ross EK, Vincenzi C, Tosti A. Videodermoscopy in the evaluation of hair and scalp disorders. J Am Acad Dermatol 2006;55:799–806.
38. Slowinska M, Rudnicka L, Schwartz RA, et al. Comma hairs: a dermatoscopic marker for tinea capitis: a rapid diagnostic method. J Am Acad Dermatol 2008; 59(Suppl 5):S77–9.
39. Duque-Estrada B, Tamler C, Pereira FBC, et al. Dermoscopic patterns of cicatricial alopecia due to discoid lupus erythematosus and lichen planopilaris. An Bras Dermatol 2009;85(2):179–83.
40. Sinclair R, Jolley D, Mallari R, et al. The reliability of horizontally sectioned scalp biopsies in the diagnosis of chronic diffuse telogen hair loss in women. J Am Acad Dermatol 2004;51:189–99.
41. Whiting DA. Diagnostic and predictive value of horizontal sections of scalp biopsy specimens in male pattern androgenetic alopecia. J Am Acad Dermatol 1993;28(5 Pt 1):755–63.
42. Van Neste DJ. Contrast enhanced phototrichogram (CE-PTG): an improved noninvasive technique for measurement of scalp hair dynamics in androgenetic

alopecia validation study with histology after transverse sectioning of scalp biopsies. Eur J Dermatol 2001;11:326–31.

43. Ueki R, Tsuboi R, Inaba Y, et al. Phototrichogram analysis of Japanese female subjects with chronic diffuse hair loss. J Investig Dermatol Symp Proc 2003;8:116–20.

44. Kantor J, Kessler LJ, Brooks DG, et al. Decreased serum ferritin is associated with alopecia in women. J Invest Dermatol 2003;121(5):985–8.

45. Messenger AG, McKillop J, Farrant P, et al. British Association of Dermatologists' guidelines for the management of alopecia areata 2012. Br J Dermatol 2012; 166(5):916–26.

46. Chartier MB, Hoss DM, Grant-kels JM. Approach to the adult female patient with diffuse non scaring alopecia. J Am Acad Dermatol 2002;47:809–19.

47. Arca E, Açikgöz G, Taştan HB, et al. An open, randomized, comparative study of oral finasteride and 5% topical minoxidil in male androgenetic alopecia. Dermatology 2004;209:117.

48. D'Amico AV, Roehrborn CG. Effect of 1 mg/day finasteride on concentrations of serum prostate-specific antigen in men with androgenic alopecia: a randomised controlled trial. Lancet Oncol 2007;8:21.

49. Avram M, Rogers N. Contemporary hair transplantation. Dermatol Surg 2009;35: 1705.

50. Blume-Peytavi U, Hillmann K, Dietz E, et al. A randomized, single-blind trial of 5% minoxidil foam once daily versus 2% minoxidil solution twice daily in the treatment of androgenetic alopecia in women. J Am Acad Dermatol 2011;65:1126.

51. Olsen EA, Messenger AG, Shapiro J, et al. Evaluation and treatment of male and female pattern hair loss. J Am Acad Dermatol 2005;52:301.

52. Vexiau P, Chaspoux C, Boudou P, et al. Effects of minoxidil 2% vs. cyproterone acetate treatment on female androgenetic alopecia: a controlled, 12-month randomized trial. Br J Dermatol 2002;146(6):992–9.

53. Rathnayake D, Sinclair R. Innovative use of spironolactone as an antiandrogen in the treatment of female pattern hair loss. Dermatol Clin 2010;28:611.

54. Avram MR. Hair transplantation for men and women. Semin Cutan Med Surg 2006;25:60.

55. Epstein JS. The treatment of female pattern hair loss and other applications of surgical hair restoration in women. Facial Plast Surg Clin North Am 2004;12:241.

56. Alkhalifah A, Alsantali A, Wang E, et al. Alopecia areata update: part II. Treatment. J Am Acad Dermatol 2010;62(2):191–202 [quiz: 203–4].

57. Gupta AK, Cooper EA. Update in antifungal therapy of dermatophytosis. Mycopathologia 2008;166:353.

58. Elewski BE, Hughey LC, Sobera JO. Fungal diseases. In: Bolognia JL, Jorizzo JL, Schaffer JV, editors. Dermatology, vol. 2, 3rd edition. Philadelphia: Elsevier Limited; 2012. p. 1251.

59. Available at: http://www.fda.gov/Drugs/DrugSafety/ucm362415.htm. Accessed July 26, 2013.

Sunburn, Thermal, and Chemical Injuries to the Skin

Aaron J. Monseau, MD[a],*, Zebula M. Reed, MD[a],
Katherine Jane Langley, MD[a], Cayce Onks, DO, MS, ATC[b,c]

KEYWORDS

- Burn • Sunburn • Chemical burn • Thermal burn • Skin injury • Frostbite

KEY POINTS

- Burns are a major cause of morbidity and mortality in the United States with an estimated 1 million injuries occurring each year, so all primary care physicians should have at least a basic knowledge of burn treatment.
- Thermal injuries can occur with both heat and cold and should be treated aggressively to avoid future disability. When children have burns, providers should have a high index of suspicion for nonaccidental trauma.
- Chemical burns are most commonly caused by acids and alkalis. Acids, except for hydrofluoric acid, cause coagulation necrosis, whereas alkalis cause liquefactive necrosis.
- Sunburns are extremely common in the United States and have been associated with both melanoma and nonmelanoma skin cancer. Protective clothing is more effective than sunscreen for most individuals.
- Acute treatment of burns should center on care of airway, breathing, and circulation, with aggressive management and early transfer to a burn center, whereas chronic management focuses on limiting disability.

Every year in the United States, approximately 450,000 burns are treated at hospitals and emergency departments with 40,000 admissions.[1] The number of burns that are treated at clinics is difficult to estimate given the lack of reliable reporting, but because simple burns are a small percentage of the 450,000, it is possible that just as many present to clinics. According to the American Burn Association, an estimated 72%

Disclosure: The authors have nothing to disclose.
[a] Department of Emergency Medicine, West Virginia University, 1 Medical Center Drive, Morgantown, WV 26506-9149, USA; [b] Department of Family & Community Medicine, Penn State Hershey Medical Center, 500 University Drive, H154, Hershey, PA 17033, USA; [c] Department of Orthopaedics and Rehabilitation, Penn State Hershey Medical Center, 500 University Drive, H154, Hershey, PA 17033, USA
* Corresponding author.
E-mail address: amonseau@hsc.wvu.edu

Prim Care Clin Office Pract 42 (2015) 591–605
http://dx.doi.org/10.1016/j.pop.2015.07.003

of burns occur in the home, whereas the next most common location is the workplace, with 9% of burns.[1]

For each burn, there are 3 areas of damage, as shown in **Fig. 1**.[2] Classic descriptions of burns refer to the depth of damage with respect to the layers of skin. **Fig. 2**B gives the basic descriptions of each degree of burn, and **Fig. 2**A indicates the body surface area that is allocated for each body part.[3] **Fig. 3** shows the level of damage for second-degree and third-degree burns.[2]

BODY SURFACE AREA

In order to best determine appropriate management of patients with burns strategies must be used for accurate estimation of body surface area involved in the burn injury. The well-established rule of 9s is often used in adults to best estimate the total percentage of body surface involved and can be found in many sources. Using this rule, the body is divided into areas of 9% or multiples of 9%. Each arm is represented by 9%, back and front of torso are each represented by 18%, each leg is represented by 18%, the head is represented by 9%, and the genital region by 1% for a total of 100%. In children and infants, the Lund and Browder burn diagrams provide a more accurate way of assessing body surface area. This tool takes into account relative percentages of areas affected by growth, allowing for larger percentages distributed to the head in infants and children. For smaller burns, the palm of an adult hand or the entire hand of a child can be used to represent approximately 1% of their body surface area.

THERMAL BURNS

Thermal injuries are a major cause of morbidity and mortality in the United States and worldwide. More than 1 million burn injuries occur annually in the United States, with most burns being preventable injuries caused by risky behavior, inattention, or improper protection.[4] The bulk of burns sustained are not admitted to the hospital for inpatient treatment, with many not seeking medical attention but self-treating at home. Children are particularly at risk for thermal injuries because of their inherent curiosity, mode of reaction, impulsiveness, and lack of experience in calculation of risks.[5] Thermal injuries can be caused by many mechanisms, such as:

- Flash injury
- Flame injury
- Scalds
- Contact and friction

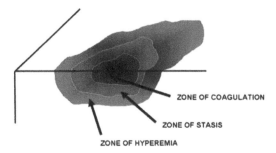

ZONE OF COAGULATION

ZONE OF STASIS

ZONE OF HYPEREMIA

Fig. 1. Three zones of damage in a burn. (*From* Gomez R, Canio LC. Management of burn wounds in the emergency department. Emerg Med Clin North Am 2007;25(1):136; with permission.)

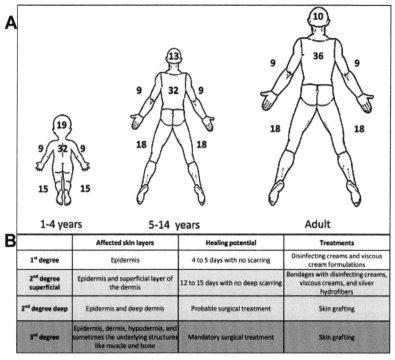

	Affected skin layers	Healing potential	Treatments
1st degree	Epidermis	4 to 5 days with no scarring	Disinfecting creams and viscous cream formulations
2nd degree superficial	Epidermis and superficial layer of the dermis	12 to 15 days with no deep scarring	Bandages with disinfecting creams, viscous creams, and silver hydrofibers
2nd degree deep	Epidermis and deep dermis	Probable surgical treatment	Skin grafting
3rd degree	Epidermis, dermis, hypodermis, and sometimes the underlying structures like muscle and bone	Mandatory surgical treatment	Skin grafting

Fig. 2. (*A*) Body surface area allocations for each body part. (*B*) Basic descriptions of each degree of burn. (*From* Deghayli L, Moufarrij S, Norberg M, et al. Insurance coverage of pediatric burns: Switzerland versus USA. Burns 2013;40(5):815; with permission.)

- Immersion and nonaccidental burns
- Frostbite

Flash injuries usually occur because of an explosion and the severity of burns depends on the type and quantity of fuel that explodes or is ignited. Flame injuries,

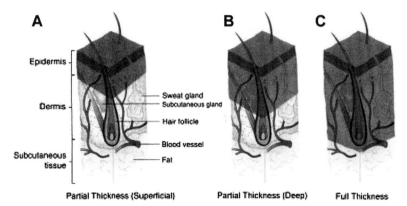

Fig. 3. Levels of damage for three classifications of second degree burns are shown for partial thickness-superficial (*A*), partial thickness-deep (*B*) and full thickness (*C*) burns. (*From* Edlich RF, Martin ML, Long WB. Thermal burns. In: Marx J, Hockberger R, Walls R, editors. Rosen's emergency medicine: concepts and clinical practice. 6th edition. St. Louis: Mosby; 2006; with permission.)

compared with flash injuries, are typically deep dermal if not full-thickness because of increased time of exposure to intense temperatures.[4] Scald burns are a typical cause of injury in the pediatric population. In children who are 1 to 4 years of age, the primary cause of burns is contact with hot surfaces or scalds. The degree of burn associated with scald injury depends on the temperature of the liquid, duration of contact, and the thickness of skin involved. The injury is typically caused by a child reaching up and pulling over a pot, kettle, or cup with hot liquid inside, with the injury pattern mainly affecting the head, neck, and torso.[6,7] Contact burns are typically associated with touching hot metal surfaces such as mufflers, stove tops, grills, or space heaters, or hot plastics, with the temperature of surface, contact duration, and thickness of skin affecting the severity of the burn. The burn pattern typically reflects the same shape and characteristics of the surface touched.

However, nonaccidental burns are common in children. The injuries tend to occur in low socioeconomic families, in crowded living conditions, and with high familial stress.[8] According to several studies, approximately 10% of physically abused children have intentional burns or scalds.[7–10] The following signs are suggestive of abuse in burns and scald injuries in children:

- Repeated burns or burns occurring in a pattern of repeated injury
- Injury incompatible with history
- Inappropriate parental response: delay in seeking treatment, blaming the child or sibling, denial that the lesion is a burn
- Site: hand, especially the back, wrist, buttocks, and feet and legs
- Type: contact burns in unusual sites, showing clear outlines of object, or scalds with clear-cut edges, and glove-and-stocking distributions.

Cigarette burns leave a circular mark that usually forms a crater and scar with a common occurrence of more than 1 burn together. Friction burns can also be a sign of child abuse. Friction occurs when something is dragged or pulled across the skin, such as carpet, rope, or cable. Friction burns typically affect the bony prominences and have broken blisters.[7] Immersion injuries are scald burns typically associated with upper and/or lower extremities in the stocking-and-glove distribution consisting of burns to the entire extremity with a well-defined border and lack of splash marks.[11] The buttocks are another common immersion site, with sparing of the portion of the buttocks pressed against the bottom of the tub or pot, called the hole-in-the-doughnut effect.[7,9–11]

Frostbite

Frostbite is another common form of thermal injury. Injury occurs when there is acute freezing of tissues when exposed to temperatures less than the freezing point of intact skin and the severity of injury depends on duration of exposure, temperature gradient at the surface of the skin, wind chill factor, and clothing.[12–15] Risk factors for developing frostbite are alcohol consumption, psychiatric illness, homelessness, and trauma involving cars, planes, or snowmobiles.[13,16] Patients at the extremes of age are more susceptible to frostbite, but it is most commonly found in adults aged 30 to 49 years.[14,17] Fingers, toes, ears, and nose are the most commonly affected sites, and damage lasts longer as the time frozen becomes longer.

The body begins a series of events as the tissue cools. The first reaction to cold exposure is vasoconstriction. Frostbite commonly has 3 major phases that produce damage: tissue freezing, hypoxia, and release of inflammatory mediators. As the time exposed increases, the body begins to have 5-minute to 10-minute cycles of vasoconstriction and vasodilation, which is a phenomenon called the hunting reaction.[12,15–17] Initially, ice crystals form in the extracellular tissue, which draws water from inside the cells into the extracellular spaces. Intracellular ice crystals then develop, causing damage to the cell membranes and causing intracellular dehydration, endothelial damage, and cell death.[17] Hypoxia results as vasoconstriction persists, leading to increased blood viscosity and stasis. The hypoxia and stasis lead to the release of inflammatory mediators. Several publications have attributed increased levels of prostaglandins PGF_2, PGE_2, and thromboxane A_2, which further propagate vasoconstriction, platelet aggregation, and blood vessel damage, causing worsening hypoxia, stasis, and cell death.[17–19] The inflammatory mediators increase during the rewarming and refreezing cycles so thawing should not be attempted until refreezing can be prevented.

Two main classifications exist for initial frostbite injuries: superficial and deep. After rewarming, a more specific frostbite classification can be used, consisting of first, second, third, and fourth degrees, which is partially determine by whether the affected tissues have permanent damage. See **Table 1** for classifications of frostbite.[12,15,20]

Chemical Burns

Chemical burns account for approximately 3% of burns, but other sources give a range of 2% to 10%.[21,22] Chemical burns occur as accidental burns at home, industrial work places, and less commonly by intentional attacks. Intentional attacks using acids and other substances are becoming more common, especially in developing countries. Women are more likely to be victims of intentional burning than men, but men are more likely to sustain accidental chemical burns.[23] The most common body areas affected are face, lower extremities, and hands, specifically the right, because of dominance.[22,23]

Chemical injuries typically have a longer exposure time than thermal injuries, which are usually caused by a short-term exposure to intense temperatures. In thermal

Table 1 Common classifications of frostbite		
Initial Classification	**Degree of Frostbite**	**Clinical Manifestations**
Superficial	First	Partial skin freezing White or yellow plaque Numbness, erythema, hyperemia No blisters Occasional skin sloughing
	Second	Full-thickness skin freezing Erythema, edema Blisters Clear or milky fluid in vesicles
Deep	Third	Full-thickness and subcutaneous freezing Hemorrhagic blisters; eschar 2 wk later Skin necrosis
	Fourth	Full-thickness skin, subcutaneous tissue, muscle, tendon, and bone freezing Initially mottled, deep red, or cyanotic Later dry, black, mummified

Data from Refs.[12,15,20]

injuries, rapid coagulation of proteins occurs because of cross-linking reactions, whereas in chemical burns protein destruction is mainly by hydrolysis reactions.[24] Chemical injuries may seem to be mild at first but as time progresses extensive damage or systemic toxicity can occur without rapid treatment.[25] The contact time of a chemical substance is correlated with the severity of burn. Multiple factors affect the severity of the chemical injury:

- Mechanism of action of chemical
- Concentration
- Quantity of agent
- Duration of skin contact, either direct or indirect
- Penetration of substance

Factors that affect the absorption of the chemical play a role in severity of injury as well:

- Body site and percentage of surface area affected
- Integrity of skin
- Nature of chemical: lipophilic, pH, concentration
- Occlusion: garments, dressings

Many different chemicals can result in injury to human skin. The most common substances resulting in injury are acids and alkalis. With the exception of hydrofluoric acid, acids release hydrogen ions and produce coagulation necrosis that results in eschar formation limiting the depth of the burn. Hydrofluoric acid causes damage similar to alkalis, resulting in tissue loss and bone destruction. Common acids that cause injury are listed in **Table 2**.[26] Alkalis join with protons and lipids to form soluble complexes and soaps that allow deeper penetration of the substances into skin, resulting in liquefactive necrosis.[25] The liquefaction loosens the tissue planes and allows the agent to continue to penetrate, causing extensive damage.[24] Other chemical agents that cause damage are desiccants and vesicants, oxidizing and reducing agents, and hydrocarbons. **Table 3** lists common chemicals and their uses.[25,27]

SUNBURN
Background

Sunburn is a common occurrence, with rates in outdoor workers as high as 50% to 80% per season.[28] Up to 80% of lifetime sun exposure takes place before the age

Table 2	
Chemical agents and their corresponding type of tissue damage	
Type of Chemical Agent	**Mechanism of Tissue Damage**
Acids	Coagulative necrosis
Alkali agents	Saponification and liquefactive necrosis
Desiccants and vesicants	Dehydration of cells through exothermic reactions, release of amines within cells
Oxidizing and reducing agents	Denaturing of proteins and direct cytotoxic effects
Hydrocarbons	Fat-dissolving corrosive injury to skin

From Druck J. Chemical burns. In: Adams JG, editor. Emergency medicine: clinical essentials. 2nd edition. Philadelphia: Saunders; 2012. p. 1595; with permission.

Table 3
Common chemicals and their uses

Chemical	Industrial Use	Domestic Use
Hydrofluoric acid	Glass etching, microchip manufacturing, germicides, dyes, fireproofing material	Rust remover
Chromic acid	Alloy production, plating, dye manufacturing	None
Sulfuric and hydrochloric acid	Refining and manufacturing reagent	Drain cleaner, lead-acid car batteries
Nitric acid	Iron and steel casting, electroplating, fertilizer manufacturing, engraving	Engraving
Carbolic acid	Synthetic manufacturing	Chemical peels, pharmaceuticals
Acetic acid	Solvents	Hair-wave neutralizer
Bleach (sodium or calcium hypochlorite	Industrial oxidizing reagent, bleach, disinfectant	Bleaching and cleaning products
Anhydrous ammonia	Fertilizers	Fertilizers
Petroleum products	Fuel, solvents, synthetic manufacturing	Fuel, solvents
Formic acid	Acrylate glue makers, cellulose formate, tanning workers	Tanning, glues
Oxalic acid	Leather tanning, blueprint paper	Leather tanning, blueprint paper
Cement (calcium oxide)	Construction	Construction
Lye (sodium hydroxide)	Manufacturing of soaps and petroleum products, paper and metal processing	Drain and oven cleaners, paint removers
Lime	Agricultural products, cement	Agricultural products, cement
White phosphorus	Munitions, pesticides, fertilizers	Fireworks, illegal methamphetamine production

Adapted from Tintinalli JE, Stapczynski JS, Ma OJ, et al. Tintinalli's emergency medicine: a comprehensive study guide. 7th edition. New York: McGraw-Hill; 2011. p. 1374–86; and Robinson EP, Chhabra AB. Hand chemical burns. J Hand Surg Am 2015;40(3):605–12.

of 18 years.[29] Skin type can commonly dictate who may be at risk for sunburn and associated morbidity as classified by the Fitzpatrick skin types:

1. Always burns, never tans.
2. Always burns, sometimes tans.
3. Sometimes burns, gradually tans.
4. Sometimes burns, tans well.
5. Rarely burns, always tans. Brown skin.[30]

Cancer Risk

Skin cancer is the most common cancer in the United States with approximately 2 million patients diagnosed every year.[31] Studies have linked skin cancer with ultraviolet radiation (UVR), which is emitted primarily through solar radiation or sunlight. The International Agency for Research on Cancer noted that there is sufficient evidence that UVR can be classified as a human carcinogen.[32]

Melanoma

The incidence of melanoma in white Americans was 27.6 per 100,000 in 2008 with approximately 70,000 cases and 8800 deaths in 2011. It is 20 times more likely in white than in African American individuals.[31] Although it is less common than basal or squamous cell cancers, it accounts for most deaths, which is why efforts have been directed toward its prevention. There is convincing evidence that incidence is strongly related to UVR.[32] Having a history of 5 or more severe sunburns in adolescence has been shown to double a person's risk for melanoma.[33] Indoor tanning is a World Health Organization group 1 carcinogen associated with melanoma and accounting for 3400 cases yearly in Europe.[34]

Nonmelanoma skin cancer

Nonmelanoma skin cancer (NMSC) is the most common malignancy, with greater than 30% of white people who live in highly exposed areas developing NMSC.[35] Evidence for NMSC suggests that risk is related to accumulation of intermittent UVR exposure in early life rather than lifetime exposure.[32] Indoor tanning has also been shown to be a significant risk factor. NMSC is often overlooked because it often does not affect survival, but it does cause significant burden on the health care system.[35]

Eye Injury

Photokeratitis is the only known acute effect of UVR on the eye.[36] This condition has been described as snowblindness, welder's flash, or sunburn of the eye, and is thought to be a painful inflammatory state that typically resolves within 48 hours. Chronic exposure of UVR has been associated with ocular melanoma with an incidence between 6 and 10 per million. In addition, there is evidence that cataracts and pterygium are associated with UVR exposure.[32]

Prevention

Sunscreen

The role of sunscreen in the prevention of melanoma is controversial. Postulated reasons for this include:

- False sense of protection.
- Inadequate application (tests for sun protection factor require a 2.0 mg/cm^2 coating and frequent application). Most consumers apply at 0.5 or 1.0 mg/cm^2
- Fair-skinned people already take more precautions.
- Difficult to study cause-and-effect relationship because melanoma occurs 10 to 50 years after sun exposure.
- Historical accounts of sunburn are inaccurate or biased.[37]

Despite these shortcomings, a recent randomized controlled trial reported that regular sunscreen application may prevent the development of melanoma for up to 10 years.[38] Current recommendations are to counsel children, adolescents, and young adults between the ages of 10 and 24 years who have fair skin to minimize their sun exposure.[31] In addition, it is suggested that counseling should include:

- Do not use sunscreen to prolong exposure to sun.
- Seek shelter if skin becomes red or uncomfortable.
- Sunscreen should be used as an adjunct to clothing, hats, and sunglasses.
- Sunscreen should provide protection against ultraviolet A and ultraviolet B.
- High-risk individuals may benefit from daily broad-spectrum sunscreen.[39]

Clothing

It is estimated that sun avoidance could reduce the number of nonmelanoma skin cancers by 80%. The National Council on Skin Cancer Prevention has recommended wearing protective clothing, hats, and sunglasses. Clothing provides ultraviolet protection factors (UPFs) that do not diminish during the day. UPFs greater than 15 are considered sun protective and factors such as darker color, tighter weave, treated fabrics, and more coverage add to the UPF.[40]

Management of Burns

Management of burns varies greatly depending on type and depth of burn, total body surface involved, and body location of burn. Although some small minor burn injuries can be managed in an outpatient setting, other more complex injuries require inpatient management or transfer to a regional burn center. Early recognition of patients who are appropriate for transfer is crucial to improving patient outcomes. The American Burn Association supported by the American College of Surgeons has developed referral criteria for regional burn centers, which can be found in **Box 1**.[41]

Box 1
Transfer criteria

Transfer criteria for burns

1. Partial-thickness burns greater than 10% total body surface area.

2. Burns that involve the face, hands, feet, genitalia, perineum, or major joints.

3. Third-degree burns in any age group.

4. Electrical burns, including lightning injury.

5. Chemical burns.

6. Inhalation injury.

7. Burn injuries in patients with preexisting medical disorders that could complicate management, prolong recovery, or affect mortality.

8. Any patient with burns and concomitant trauma (such as fracture) when the burn injury poses the greatest risk of mortality and morbidity. If the trauma poses the greater immediate risk, the patient's condition may be stabilized initially in a trauma center before transfer to a burn center. Physician judgment is necessary in such situations and should be in concert with the regional medical control plan and triage protocols.

9. Burns in children: children with burns should be transferred to a burn center verified to treat children. In the absence of a regional pediatric burn center, an adult burn center may serve as a second option for the management of pediatric burns.

10. Burn injury in patients who require special social, emotional, or rehabilitative intervention.

(*From* ACS Committee on Trauma. Resources for optimal care of the injured patient committee on trauma. American College of Surgeons; 2014. p. 100–2)

Burn centers help provide optimal care to patients with complex burns. According to the most recent data from the 2013 National Burn Repository Annual Report, there are currently 63 American Burn Association verified centers and 125 designated burn care centers across the United States.[42] It has been well-documented that patients with complex burns greatly benefit from a well-integrated multidisciplinary team providing their care.[43–45] Team members often include burn surgeons, nurses, anesthesiologists, respiratory therapists, occupational and physical therapists, dieticians, and psychosocial experts.[44] These members work closely together in order to provide a centralized approach to care. The success of improvement in burn care has been reflected in the most recent National Burn Repository data from 2013, which show that overall mortality for women decreased 2% to 3.6% in 2012 from 5.6% in 2003, and for men decreased to 2.6% from 3.5%.[42]

ACUTE MANAGEMENT

Burn incidents can happen anywhere, at any time, and vary greatly in the extent of injury. Basic first aid at the time of initial injury can help minimize morbidity associated with burn injury.[46] For most burns, application of cool water immediately following burn injury may be beneficial in both healing outcomes and providing analgesia to the area.[47] Patients with minor injury can often be managed in an outpatient setting. Initial management in an outpatient setting includes analgesia, assessment of size and depth of wound, application of clean and dry dressing, confirming updated tetanus immunization, and plan for reevaluation in 24 to 48 hours following injury.[47]

Patients with moderate to severe burns require more intensive evaluation and resuscitative measures. During initial emergency department resuscitation and stabilization this patient population is treated using advanced trauma life support strategies. Initial evaluation centers on the primary survey. The first step is evaluation of the airway and consideration of intubation if there is concern for inhalation injury or airway compromise.[48] The remainder of the primary survey is performed, including breathing, circulation, disability, and exposure, ensuring that all have been adequately addressed. During the secondary survey, further assessment of the extent of the burn injury as well as an estimate of body surface area injured is determined. Following evaluation of the burn injury, the involved area should be protected from contamination using clean, dry linens.[46] During assessment of patients with burn injuries clinicians must remember to provide adequate fluid resuscitation and appropriate analgesia, and confirm updated tetanus status. Once the patient is stabilized, a determination can be made regarding the need to transfer to a regional burn center for further management.

SPECIAL CONSIDERATION FOR SPECIFIC BURN SITES
Facial Burns

During evaluation of a patient with facial burns it is important to remember airway management, as previously discussed. With burns to the head and neck, ongoing reevaluation of airway is crucial in management. Although patients may be able to support their own airways during initial assessment, external pressure on the airway caused by swelling and edema of the face and neck may quickly compromise the airway. In patients with facial burns, early intubation is often beneficial.[49]

Ocular Burns

Thermal burns of the face require special attention to be paid to the eye. A detailed examination of the globe early in care is crucial because edema may develop rapidly and prevent close examination later in the course of care. Corneal burns should be noted and appropriate eye drops administered.[49]

Chemical Burns of the Face and Eye

As discussed earlier, most chemical burns are caused by alkaline and acidic agents. These exposures often happen in industrial, laboratory, or construction settings. Immediately following exposure copious water irrigation to the affected area should be used.[49,50] For ocular injuries, irrigation with normal saline or lactated Ringer solution with volumes up to 20 L may be required to change pH levels. It is important to obtain pH testing of the eye early in management and following irrigation in order to ensure that pH has neutralized back to physiologic levels.[50] Following irrigation, a detailed ocular examination should be performed to determine the extent of injury. Emergent ophthalmologic consultation is likely to be necessary. Acute treatment centers on topical antibiotics, cycloplegic agents, and antiglaucoma therapy; topical steroids may also be used to help control inflammation.[50]

Hand Burns

Hand burns represent most isolated burn injuries as well as part of larger burn injuries.[51] The outcomes of these injuries can greatly affect patients' ability to perform activities of daily living. Complications from hand burns include vascular compromise, contractures, deformities, and significant edema.[52] Appropriate initial management of these burns can greatly limit complications and depends on depth of burn injury. All finger injuries benefit from individual wound dressing, splinting in position of function, and early range of motion exercises.[52] Superficial and partial-thickness burns are often managed with local wound care, whereas deeper burns may require surgical intervention.[51]

Immersion Burns

Liquid immersion burns can occur accidentally as a fall into liquid or intentionally as a child is placed into a hot liquid.[9] The injury patterns for accidental versus intentional immersion burns are distinctive. In the case of an accidental injury, spill and splash patterns are often present with indistinct borders and variable depths of injury. The history of this injury is often consistent with burn pattern and may involve children pulling hot liquid onto themselves or falling into hot liquid. In the case of intentional injury, there often are burns with distinctive borders of uniform depth. Skin-fold sparing can be seen and distribution of injury may be in a stocking-glove pattern. It is estimated that intentional burns associated with suspected or known abuse make up approximately 10% of pediatric burn injuries.[53] If there is concern for intentional injury, the provider must evaluate for additional injuries associated with abuse as well as report concern to appropriate authorities.

TREATMENT OF BURNS
Fluid Resuscitation

Moderate to severe burn injuries can lead to hypovolemic shock.[43] Early and effective fluid resuscitation is critical in the management of this population of patients with burns. Although multiple strategies and formulas have been developed, the most commonly accepted formula is the Parkland formula. The Parkland formula, developed by Dr Charles Baxter in the 1960s, uses the patient's body weight in kilograms and percentage body surface burned to estimate the amount of fluid resuscitation a patient requires immediately following a burn injury.

Parkland equation:

4 mL × weight (kg) × percentage of body surface area burned = milliliters of crystalloid fluid in first 24 hours

Give half of the resuscitative fluids in the first 8 hours from the time of the burn.
Give the second half of the resuscitative fluids over the subsequent 16 hours.

Note that this formula should only be used to help guide resuscitative management because some experts have indicated that the Parkland equation may overhydrate patients. Adjustments for individual patients should be made based on overall clinical picture as well as type of burn injury. Often, adequate urinary output (0.1 mg/kg/h), as well as laboratory markers, are followed to help further guide resuscitative management.[43,45] However, adequate burn shock resuscitation commonly requires an experienced burn team in order to reduce the complications from both over-resuscitation and under-resuscitation.[43]

COMPARTMENT SYNDROME AND CIRCUMFERENTIAL BURNS

Third-degree and deep second-degree circumferential and near-circumferential burns are at high risk for complications from compartment syndrome. Compartment syndrome is defined as pressures greater than 30 mm Hg that lead to critical compromise of perfusion to the limb.[54] Escharotomy should be considered early in patients with circumferential burns to limbs in order to prevent compartment syndrome.[48,52] Escharotomy should also be considered in patients with deep or circumferential burns to neck or chest in order to prevent airway compromise.[49,52] The procedure entails making an incision along escharotomy lines through the eschar in order to expose the fatty tissue below. If escharotomy is not performed early enough and compartment syndrome does develop, a fasciotomy should be considered. Fasciotomy to treat acute compartment syndrome is considered to be a limb-saving procedure. A fasciotomy is performed by making an incision that extends into the fascia and thus relieving the pressure in the compartment, which subsequently allows return of blood flow to the compartment.[48]

TOPICAL AND SYSTEMIC TREATMENTS

Topical and systemic treatment of burns depend on degree of burns, location of burns, and concerns for contamination of burn. The early treatment of burns centers on moist wound healing to help decrease cellular dehydration and promote reepithelialization.[55] These environments can be created using topical agents or use of occlusive dressings. Superficial burns heal within a week and may only require topical hydrating lotions or aloe vera for treatment. These minor wounds often only require topical antibiotics if there is concern for a contaminated wound. Superficial partial-thickness and deep partial-thickness wounds require longer healing times and are often dressed with topical antibacterials or topical antimicrobial-containing substances such as silver sulfadiazine.[47] Newer biosynthetic dressings, silver-containing dressings, and silicon-coated dressings showed some advantages compared with silver sulfadiazine in a 2008 Cochrane Review, and their use should be considered.[56] There is no role for systemic prophylactic antibiotics in patients with burns.[43,53]

OUTCOMES OF BURN INJURY

Outcomes of burn injury depend on many variables, including total body surface area involved, type of injury, location of injury, age of patient, and associated injuries. Small superficial wounds often heal in 7 days and do not show scarring. Superficial partial-thickness wounds often heal in 7 to 14 days and carry a low risk for scarring but may show some pigmentation changes. Deep partial wounds take greater than 21 days for healing and are at greatest risk for hypertrophic scarring.[47] Complications from scarring range from aesthetic to functional problems. In patients with persistent stiffness or scarring over joints, surgical scar revisions may be required to improve function.

According to the National Burn Repository data from 2013, men made up 69% of all patients with burns, with children less than the age of 5 years accounting for 20% of the cases and adults more than the age of 60 years accounting for 12% of the cases. Of all burns reported, 73% involved less than 10% of the total body surface area and carried a mortality of 0.6% compared with mortality for all cases of 3.4%. These data also show that the mortality for women with burn injuries is higher than for men: 3.6%–2.6% respectively. Risk of death from burn injury increases with advancing age and larger burn size. In thermal burn, the presence of concomitant inhalation injury also greatly increases the likelihood of death.[42]

SUMMARY

Sunburn, thermal, and chemical injuries to skin are a significant cause of morbidity and mortality in the United States and around the world. Proper acute care of these injuries is important for all health care providers because they can present at any time. Early consultation with a burn center may prove helpful because burn centers offer recommendations on management, transfer, or follow-up. When providing care for burns, clinicians must always remember to first care for airway, breathing, and circulation because these may quickly be threatened with significant burns.

REFERENCES

1. Burn incidence and treatment in the United States: 2013 fact sheet. American Burn Association. Available at: http://ameriburn.org/resources_factsheet.php. Accessed April 4, 2015.
2. Gomez R, Canio LC. Management of burn wounds in the emergency department. Emerg Med Clin North Am 2007;25(1):135–46.
3. Deghayli L, Moufarrij S, Norberg M, et al. Insurance coverage of pediatric burns: Switzerland versus USA. Burns 2013;40(5):814–25.
4. Keck M, Herndon DH, Kamolz LP, et al. Pathophysiology of burns. Wien Med Wochenschr 2009;159:327–36.
5. Lindblad BE, Terkelsen CJ. Domestic burns among children. Burns 1990;16(4): 254–6.
6. Drago DA. Kitchen scalds and thermal burns in children five years and younger. Pediatrics 2005;115:10.
7. Hobbs CJ. ABC of child abuse. Burns and scalds. BMJ 1989;298:1302–5.
8. Hansbrough JF, Hansbrough W. Pediatric burns. Pediatr Rev 1999;20:117–23.
9. Toon MH, Maybauer DM, Arceneaux LL, et al. Children with burn injuries-assessment of trauma, neglect, violence and abuse. J Inj Violence Res 2011; 3(2):98–110.
10. Stratman E, Melski J. Scald abuse. Arch Dermatol 2002;138:318–20.
11. Peck MD, Priolo-Kapel D. Child abuse by burning: a review of the literature and an algorithm for medical investigations. J Trauma 2002;53(5):1013–22.
12. Murphy JV, Banwell PE, Roberts AH, et al. Frostbite: pathogenesis and treatment. J Trauma Inj Infect Crit Care 2000;48(1):171–8.

13. Valnicek SM, Chasmar LR, Clapson JB. Frostbite in the prairies: a 12-year review. Plast Reconstr Surg 1993;92(4):633–41.
14. Handford C, Buxton P, Russell K, et al. Frostbite: a practical approach to hospital management. Extrem Physiol Med 2014;3:7.
15. Imray C, Grieve A, Dhillon S, et al. Cold damage to the extremities: frostbite and non-freezing cold injuries. Postgrad Med J 2009;85:481–8.
16. Britt LD, Dascombe WH, Rodriguez A. New horizons in management of hypothermia and frostbite injury. Surg Clin North Am 1991;71(2):345–70.
17. Reamy BV. Frostbite: review and current concepts. J Am Board Fam Pract 1998; 11(1):34–40.
18. Heggers JP, Robson MC, Manavalen K, et al. Experimental and clinical observations on frostbite. Ann Emerg Med 1987;16(9):1056–62.
19. Bracker MD. Environmental and thermal injury. Clin Sports Med 1992;11(2): 419–36.
20. McIntosh SE, Hamonko M, Freer L, et al. Wilderness medical society practice guidelines for the prevention and treatment of frostbite. Wilderness Environ Med 2011;22:156–66.
21. D'Cruz R, Pang TC, Harvey JG, et al. Chemical burns in children: aetiology and prevention. Burns 2015;41(4):764–9.
22. Hardwicke J, Hunter T, Staruch R, et al. Chemical burns-an historical comparison and review of the literature. Burns 2012;38:383–7.
23. Das KK, Olga L, Peck M, et al. Management of acid burns: experience from Bangladesh. Burns 2015;41:484–92.
24. Palao R, Monge I, Ruiz M, et al. Chemical burns: pathophysiology and treatment. Burns 2010;36(3):295–304.
25. Tintinalli JE, Stapczynski JS, Ma OJ, et al. Tintinalli's emergency medicine: a comprehensive study guide. 7th edition. New York: McGraw-Hill; 2011. p. 1374–86.
26. Druck J. Chemical Burns. In: Adams JG, editor. Emergency medicine: clinical essentials. 2nd edition. Philadelphia: Saunders; 2012. p. 1594–7.
27. Robinson EP, Chhabra AB. Hand chemical burns. J Hand Surg Am 2015;40(3): 605–12.
28. Reinau D, Weiss M, Meier CR, et al. Outdoor workers' sun-related knowledge, attitudes and protective behaviours: a systematic review of cross-sectional and interventional studies. Br J Dermatol 2013;168(5):928–40.
29. Quatrano NA, Dinulos JG. Current principles of sunscreen use in children. Curr Opin Pediatr 2013;25:122–9. United States.
30. Baron ED, Suggs AK. Introduction to photobiology. Dermatol Clin 2014;32(3): 255–66, vii.
31. Moyer VA. Behavioral counseling to prevent skin cancer: U.S. Preventive Services Task Force recommendation statement. Ann Intern Med 2012;157:59–65. United States.
32. Gallagher RP, Lee TK. Adverse effects of ultraviolet radiation: a brief review. Prog Biophys Mol Biol 2006;92:119–31. United Kingdom.
33. Gilchrest BA, Eller MS, Geller AC, et al. The pathogenesis of melanoma induced by ultraviolet radiation. N Engl J Med 1999;340(17):1341–8.
34. Wehner MR, Chren MM, Nameth D, et al. International prevalence of indoor tanning: a systematic review and meta-analysis. JAMA Dermatol 2014;150: 390–400. United States.
35. Wehner MR, Shive ML, Chren MM, et al. Indoor tanning and non-melanoma skin cancer: systematic review and meta-analysis. BMJ 2012;345:e5909.

36. Young AR. Acute effects of UVR on human eyes and skin. Prog Biophys Mol Biol 2006;92:80–5. United Kingdom.
37. Mulliken JS, Russak JE, Rigel DS. The effect of sunscreen on melanoma risk. Dermatol Clin 2012;30:369–76. United States: Elsevier Inc.
38. Green AC, Williams GM, Logan V, et al. Reduced melanoma after regular sunscreen use: randomized trial follow-up. J Clin Oncol 2011;29:257–63. United States.
39. Planta MB. Sunscreen and melanoma: is our prevention message correct? J Am Board Fam Med 2011;24:735–9. United States.
40. Balk SJ. Ultraviolet radiation: a hazard to children and adolescents. Pediatrics 2011;127:e791–817. United States.
41. Rotondo MF, Cribari C, Smith RS. Resources for optimal care of the injured patient committee on trauma. Chicago (IL): American College of Surgeons; 2014. p. 100–2.
42. Bessey PQ, Lentz CW, Edelman LS, et al. American Burn Association: National Burn Repository 2013 report. Available at: http://www.ameriburn.org/2013NBRAnnualReport.pdf. Accessed August 18, 2014.
43. Snell JA, Loh NW, Mahambrey T, et al. Clinical review: the critical care management of the burn patient. Crit Care 2013;17:241.
44. Al-Mousawi AM, Mecott-Rivera GA, Jeschke MG, et al. Burn teams and burn centers: the importance of a comprehensive team approach to burn care. Clin Plast Surg 2009;36(4):547–54.
45. Dries DJ. Management of burn injuries – recent developments in resuscitation, infection control and outcomes research. Scand J Trauma Resusc Emerg Med 2009;17:14.
46. Shrivastava P, Goel A. Pre-hospital care in burn injury. Indian J Plast Surg 2010; 43(Suppl):S15–22.
47. Cleland H. Thermal burns - assessment and acute management in the general practice setting. Aust Fam Physician 2012;41(6):372–5.
48. Alharbi Z, Piatkowski A, Dembinski R, et al. Treatment of burns in the first 24 hours: simple and practice guide by answering 10 questions in a step-by-step form. World J Emerg Surg 2012;7:13.
49. Burd A. Burns: treatment and outcomes. Semin Plast Surg 2010;24:262–80.
50. Singh P, Tyagi M, Kumar Y, et al. Ocular chemical injuries and their management. Oman J Ophthalmol 2013;6(2):83–6.
51. Kowalske KJ, Greenhalgh DG, Ward SR. Hand burns. J Burn Care Res 2007; 28(4):607–10.
52. Bilwank PK. Unfavourable results in acute burn management. Indian J Plast Surg 2013;46(2):428–33.
53. Maguire S, Moynihan S, Mann M, et al. A systematic review of the features that indicate intentional scalds in children. Burns 2008;34:1072–81.
54. Coban YK. Rhabdomyolysis, compartment syndrome and thermal injury. World J Crit Care Med 2014;3(1):1–7.
55. Singer AJ, Dagum AB. Current management of acute cutaneous wounds. N Engl J Med 2008;359:1037–46.
56. Wasiak J, Cleland H, Campbell F, et al. Dressings for superficial and partial thickness burns. Cochrane Database Syst Rev 2013;(3):CD002106.

Dermatologic Manifestations of Systemic Diseases

Maryn Anne Valdez, MD[a], Nwamaka Isamah, MD[a],*,
Rebecca M. Northway, MD[b]

KEYWORDS

- Dermatology • Systemic disease • Skin findings • Gastrointestinal conditions
- Rheumatologic conditions

KEY POINTS

- Certain dermatologic conditions can be associated with systemic illness, and patients may present initially with a dermatologic complaint; therefore, the primary care physician should be familiar with the dermatologic sequela of systemic diseases.
- Initial evaluation almost always involves various laboratory studies.
- Treatment is specific to the particular underlying diagnosis and can include surveillance with clinical evaluations and laboratory monitoring, pharmacotherapy with topical or oral medications such as steroids or immune modulators, and directed treatment of the underlying systemic condition.
- Consultation with various subspecialists, such as Dermatology, Rheumatology, and Gastroenterology, may be warranted for particular conditions that require further management.

PYODERMA GANGRENOSUM

Definition

Pyoderma gangrenosum (PG) is a rare but serious noninfectious ulceration of the skin with unknown cause. It is characterized by painful cutaneous ulcerations with muco-purulent and sometimes hemorrhagic exudate. Although the underlying cause is poorly understood, the formation of PG has been linked to the dysregulation of the

Disclosure Statement: Authors have nothing to disclose.
[a] Penn State Hershey Family and Community Medicine Residency Program, Department of Family Medicine, Penn State Milton S. Hershey Medical Center, 500 University Drive, H154, PO Box 850, Hershey, PA 17033-0850, USA; [b] Internal Medicine-Pediatrics, University of Michigan Medical Hospital, University of Michigan, 1500 East Medical Center Drive, Ann Arbor, MI 48105, USA
* Corresponding author.
E-mail address: nisamah@hmc.psu.edu

immune system. More than half of individuals affected have other associated systemic diseases such as inflammatory bowel disease (IBD) and rheumatoid disease. In approximately 30% of patients affected, new ulcerations are typically secondary to pathergy formation of ulcers following injury or trauma to the skin. PG can also affect other organ systems such as the central nervous system, lymph nodes, gastrointestinal (GI) tract, liver, and spleen.[1–3]

Epidemiology

PG occurs predominantly among women. The peak of incidence is typically within the ages of 20 and 50 years with a general incidence estimated between 3 to 10 per million per year.[3,4]

Clinical Presentation

Initially, individuals often present with symptoms of generalized malaise such as fevers, arthralgias, and myalgias. The lesion itself usually starts as small pustules and within days grows rapidly, forming an open sore with tissue necrosis. Other associated symptoms include a strong sensation of pain and malodor secondary to infection. Although these ulcers may affect any part of the skin, it is most commonly seen over the lower extremities. The classic appearance of pyoderma gangrenosa is a deep ulcer with well-defined violaceous borders (**Fig. 1**). Edema, erythema, and induration of the surrounding tissue are often present as well.[2,3]

Differential Diagnosis

- Cutaneous vasculitis
- Malignancy
- Other skin infections

Associated Gastrointestinal Conditions

Approximately 50% cases are associated with some form of systemic diseases and more commonly GI conditions such as IBD.[2,5]

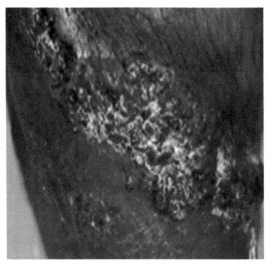

Fig. 1. Pyoderma gangrenosa. (*Courtesy of* Freire da Silva S. Dermatology Atlas. Available at: http://www.atlasdermatologico.com.br/index.jsf. Accessed April 25, 2015.)

Diagnosis

Although PD is usually diagnosed clinically after a comprehensive history and physical examination, laboratory evaluation and a skin biopsy are done to exclude all other causes of comparable ulcerations. A colonoscopy may also be performed to assess for associated IBD.[2,5]

Laboratory evaluation should include the following:
- Complete blood count (CBC)
- Comprehensive metabolic panel
- Liver function test
- Hepatitis profile
- Coagulation studies
- Anti-neutrophilic cytoplasmic antibody (ANCA) test
- Wound culture

Treatment

Although consultation with specialists is often required to guide therapy, the mainstay of treatment is with immunosuppressive therapy. Systemic corticosteroids and cyclosporine are the 2 main first-line agents. Alternative treatment options include mycophenolate mofetil, tacrolimus, infliximab, and plasmapheresis.[2] Additional measures to promote wound healing include medical or surgical debridement, occlusive dressing, adequate nutrition, and treatment of superimposed infection.

Prognosis

Although unpredictable, prognosis is generally good. PG ulcers usually parallel activity and severity of bowel disease.[1,3]

ERYTHEMA NODOSUM
Definition

Erythema nodosum (EN) is an inflammatory condition within the subcutaneous layer of the skin. More often than not, it indicates an underlying infection or inflammation.

Epidemiology

The incidence of EN is 1 to 5 of 100,000 occurring most often in young adults, with a higher female to male ratio.[6,7]

Clinical Presentation

Several patients presenting with EN have a history of recent streptococcal infection. However, a history of GI discomfort and changes in bowel pattern, most notably diarrhea, is usually suggestive of an associated inflammatory bowel disorder. Prodromal symptoms such as fever, weight loss, malaise, upper respiratory symptoms, arthritis, and arthralgia may precede skin eruption. During the actual eruptive phase, systemic symptoms comprising fever, abdominal pain, vomiting, and diarrhea may also be present.[7]

Lesions of erythema nodosum

The classic presentation of EN is the development of sudden extremely tender, warm, erythematous subcutaneous nodules, 1 to 10 cm in diameter, with poorly defined edges usually located on the pretibial surfaces. Other body surfaces such as the forearms, thighs, trunk, head, or neck may also be affected (**Fig. 2**). Within 2 to 3 weeks of onset, lesions subsequently evolve and change color to look like a bruise with a

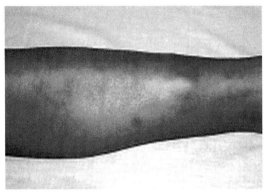

Fig. 2. Erythema nodosum involving the anterior aspect of the lower extremities. (*Courtesy of* Freire da Silva S. Dermatology Atlas. Available at: http://www.atlasdermatologico.com.br/index.jsf. Accessed April 25, 2015.)

yellowish purple discoloration. Eventually, lesions fade within 1 to 2 months of onset.[6–10]

Differential Diagnosis

- Traumatic bruises
- Superficial thrombophlebitis
- Subcutaneous fat necrosis
- Insect bite
- Acute urticarial reaction
- Sarcoidosis

Associated Gastrointestinal Conditions

Associated GI conditions include ulcerative colitis and Crohn disease.

Diagnosis

Diagnostic evaluation after a thorough history and physical examination should include laboratory tests, evaluation of IBD and skin biopsy.

Laboratory evaluation

- Throat culture
- Anti-streptolysin O titer
- Tuberculosis skin test
- Inflammatory markers: CBC, erythrocyte sedimentation rate (ESR), C-reactive protein (CRP)

Evaluation of inflammatory bowel disease

- Laboratory markers: CBC, ESR, CRP, ANCA test
- Diagnostic studies: computed tomography, colonoscopy

Deep incisional or excisional skin biopsy

- Histopathology reveals septal panniculitis with neutrophilic infiltration around proliferating capillaries. Actinic granulomas are also characteristic findings.[7,9]

Treatment

Although most cases of EN resolve spontaneously, therapy is aimed at treatment of the underlying cause. In cases with mild skin involvement, conservative treatment with bed rest, leg elevation to relieve edema, and nonsteroidal anti-inflammatory drugs (NSAIDs) is usually recommended. However, severe cases with extensive cutaneous involvement usually require a short course of systemic corticosteroids. Immunosuppressive therapy such as colchicine, hydroquinolone, or oral potassium iodide may also be considered.[7–11]

NSAIDs should be avoided when treating EN secondary to Crohn disease as this may precipitate a flare-up.[7]

Prognosis

EN is typically self-limited with lesions spontaneously resolving within 1 to 2 months from onset. Lesions that fail to resolve usually indicate uncontrolled IBD.[6,7]

APTHOUS STOMATITIS
Definition

Apthous stomatitis, also known as canker sore, is a common condition with an unknown cause. It is characterized as a recurrent shallow and painful oral mucosal ulcer. Although usually a self-limited condition that resolves within 7 to 10 days of onset, larger lesions can last anywhere from weeks to months.[6,10,12,13]

Epidemiology

Apthous stomatitis is a common condition encountered by both physicians and dentists. It affects 20% to 60% of the general population and occurs more commonly among the young adult population.[6,10,12,13]

Clinical Presentation

Individuals affected with canker sores usually present with approximately 2- to 5-mm, single or multiple, round, punched-out ulcers with yellow or gray necrotic surface surrounded by erythema (**Fig. 3**). The most common locations are within the buccal and

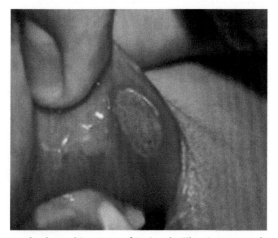

Fig. 3. Recurrent mouth ulcers. (*Courtesy of* Freire da Silva S. Dermatology Atlas. Available at: http://www.atlasdermatologico.com.br/index.jsf. Accessed April 25, 2015.)

labial mucosa. Other common locations within the oral cavity include the gingiva, soft palate, floor of the mouth, and the surface of the tongue.[6,10,12,13]

Differential Diagnosis

- Herpes simplex virus (HSV) infection
- Behçet disease
- Hand-foot-and-mouth disease
- Allergic or irritant contact dermatitis

Associated Gastrointestinal Conditions

IBD is an associated condition.

Diagnosis

In addition to a thorough history and physical examination, laboratory evaluation can be useful in identifying underlying potential causes.

- Laboratory evaluation should include CBC, ESR, iron panel, vitamin B_6, and vitamin B_{12}.
- Tzanck smear and viral culture should be considered to exclude HSV infection.
- Although biopsy of the lesion is not diagnostic, it becomes a useful tool in evaluating nonhealing ulcers when an infectious or malignant process is questioned.
- If there is suspicion of GI pathology, additional diagnostic measures such as serologic testing for antinuclear antibodies (ANA) or imaging with colonoscopy should be used.

Treatment

Therapeutic intervention is based on the severity of lesions and association with other disease processes (**Fig. 4**).

Prognosis

Spontaneous resolution of minor lesions is usually achieved within 2 weeks, whereas larger ulcerations may take up to 6 weeks to heal completely. Recurrences are common, but resolution occurs quickly once remission is achieved.[6]

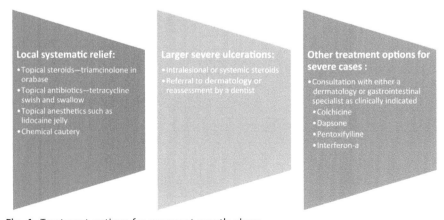

Fig. 4. Treatment options for recurrent mouth ulcers.

DERMATITIS HERPETIFORMIS
Definition

Dermatitis herpetiformis (DH) is an autoimmune disease with cutaneous manifestations linked to gluten sensitivity and most notably Celiac disease. Cutaneous deposits of IgA class of antibodies are diagnostic.[14–16]

Epidemiology

DH usually occurs during early adult life, with a higher incidence in men. The pathogenic mechanism underlying DH is multifactorial, with components of genetic, environmental, and autoimmune involvement.[14,17]

Clinical Presentation

Presentation includes intensely pruritic group of erythematous papules, vesicles, and urticarial plaques classically distributed symmetrically over the scalp, shoulders, elbow, knees, and buttocks (**Fig. 5**).[6,17]

Differential Diagnosis

- Eczema
- Papular urticaria
- Erythema multiforme
- HSV infection
- Scabies

Associated Gastrointestinal Condition

Celiac disease is the associated GI condition.

Diagnosis

In addition to clinical findings, laboratory studies including serology and tissue histopathology of skin biopsies can be performed to aid in obtaining a definitive diagnosis. Examples of such laboratory markers include IgA tissue transglutaminase.[16] Direct immunofluorescence of lesional and perilesional biopsy tissue has demonstrated

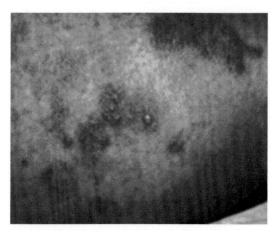

Fig. 5. Erythematous papulovesicular patches of dermatitis herpetiformis. (*Courtesy of* Freire da Silva S. Dermatology Atlas. Available at: http://www.atlasdermatologico.com. br/index.jsf. Accessed April 25, 2015.)

granular deposits of IgA within the dermal to epidermal junction.[6,17–19] A referral to a gastroenterologist may be necessary for a more invasive diagnostic workup, such as a small-bowel biopsy.

Treatment

A gluten-free diet has been shown to treat both the rash and enteropathy in cases of gluten-sensitive enteropathy. Topical steroids may also be used for symptomatic relief. Patients may be referred to the appropriate specialists for additional treatment options with immunosuppressive therapy such as dapsone and sulfasalazine.[6,14,18,20]

Prognosis

DH clears rapidly after appropriate treatment. However, continued treatment is usually necessary as lesions recur with cessation of treatment. Remission is possible with strict gluten-free diet in the cases of gluten-sensitive enteropathy.[6,14] Untreated patients with DH should be routinely monitored for malabsorption and possible development of lymphomas.[21]

LICHEN PLANUS
Definition

Lichen planus (LP) is an inflammatory disorder of the skin and mucous membrane with an unknown cause. Onset may be quick or gradual. Pruritus is a common presenting complaint. LP is neither an infectious disease nor a type of cancer. Lesions can affect the skin, hair, nails, and mucous membranes.[22]

Epidemiology

LP is uncommon but not rare and affects approximately 0.4% to 4% of the general population within the ages of 30 and 60 years. Although it affects both men and women, slight variations may exist when comparing the prevalence of cutaneous and oral LP.[23] There are also documented cases of LP in the pediatric population, although infrequently, and presentation is often atypical.[24]

Clinical Features

The lesions of LP are usually characterized as purple flat-topped violaceous papules most commonly affecting the wrists, ankles, and extremities (**Figs. 6** and **7**).[25]

Differential Diagnosis

- Psoriasis
- Eczema
- Pityriasis rosea
- Discoid lupus erythematosus
- Insect bite
- Drug eruption
- Secondary syphilis
- Tinea corporis
- Graft-versus-host disease
- Differential diagnosis for LP involving the mucous membrane include
  - Leukoplakia
  - Candidiasis
  - Secondary syphilis
  - Bite trauma

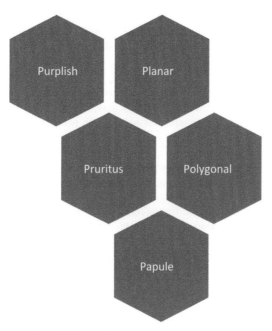

Fig. 6. The 5 P's description of lichen planus.

Associated Gastrointestinal Condition

Hepatitis C is the associated GI condition.

Diagnosis

Diagnosis is usually based on clinical findings. In addition to the classic 5 P's, findings of a superimposed reticulated white scale known as Wickham striae may be visible on close inspection or on dermascopic examination of the skin.[6,22]

A skin biopsy should be performed when in doubt and to confirm diagnosis. A characteristic saw tooth pattern of epidermal hyperplasia, hyperkeratosis, and thickened granular cell layer; degeneration of the basal cell layer; necrotic basal cells; and an intense bandlike inflammatory infiltrate at the dermal-epidermal junction are usually visualized on histopathology.[6,22,23,26]

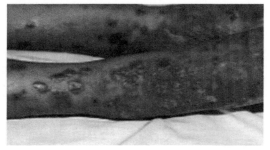

Fig. 7. Lesions of lichen planus. (*Courtesy of* Freire da Silva S. Dermatology Atlas. Available at: http://www.atlasdermatologico.com.br/index.jsf. Accessed April 25, 2015.)

Additional laboratory studies such as liver function tests and hepatitis C screening with anti-hepatitis C virus antibody testing followed by polymerase chain reaction testing should also be performed to assess for underlying viremia.[22]

Treatment

Although spontaneous resolution of lesions may be achieved within 1 to 2 years of onset and a wide array of treatment options exists, response to treatment is challenging and sometimes unsuccessful, especially with oral LP.

Cutaneous lichen planus

- First-line treatment involves high-potency topical corticosteroids.
- Severe, widespread disease is treated with oral corticosteroid such as prednisone.
- Other treatment modalities for severe cases include aciretin, sulfasalazine, cyclosporine, mycophenolate mofetil, metronidazole, griseofulvin, and phototherapy.[22,27–34]
- A dermatology referral may be necessary, especially with more severe cutaneous manifestations.

Oral lichen planus

- A consultation with a dermatology specialist is usually necessary for treatment.
- First-line treatment includes high-potency topical steroids (clobetasol, fluocinonide).
- Topical calcineurin inhibitors such as tacrolimus and pimecrolimus may be used for lesions unresponsive to topical steroids.[22]
- Severe disease is treated with oral corticosteroids.
- Other treatment options include mycophenolate mofetil, cyclosporine, methotrexate (MTX), griseofulvin, retinoids, and levamisole.[22,34–36]

Other treatment modalities

- Topical aloe vera[22]
- Antibiotics such as dapsone in the pediatric population[24,25]

Prognosis

Lesions may resolve spontaneously within 1 to 2 years. However, a more chronic and prolonged clinical course may be seen with mucosal involvement. Recurrences are still common even with treatment.[6,23,37]

ACUTE CUTANEOUS LUPUS FROM SYSTEMIC LUPUS ERYTHEMATOSUS
Definition

Systemic lupus erythematosus (SLE) is a chronic inflammatory and autoimmune disease that can affect the skin, joints, kidneys, lungs, nervous system, and multiple other organs of the body. Immunologic abnormalities, particularly the production of ANA, are a prominent feature of the disease. Anti-Smith and anti-dsDNA antibodies are also specific to the disease.[38–40]

Many types of skin lesions can occur in SLE. Skin manifestation can occur alone or with systemic involvement or as discoid skin manifestations, which are considered a separate entity. The malar rash or butterfly rash is classically associated with acute cutaneous SLE.

Epidemiology

The prevalence of SLE in the population is 20 to 150 cases per 100,000, with women outnumbering men 6 to 9 times. The prevalence among Asians, African Americans, and Hispanics is higher than in persons of European descent. The incidence is highest in women of childbearing age. In SLE, 26.4% of the time the malar rash is one of the manifestations of the disease, only surpassed by arthralgia, seen in 41% of patients.[38,40,41]

Clinical Presentation

The cutaneous disease is characterized by superficial, widespread, nonpruritic, telangiectasia, nonscarring, and erythematous plaques and skin lesions. Areas of involvement can include, but are not limited to, the face, neck, and upper and extensor surfaces of arms, particularly areas of the body exposed to the sun. Disease manifestations can be exacerbated by exposure to sun. Fine scaling on the surface of the skin may be seen without atrophy.

The classic butterfly rash, over the malar area with sparing of the nasal area, is present only in 10% to 40% of people (**Fig. 8**). Bullae, purpura, subcutaneous nodules, and discoid lesions may also be seen in SLE.[38,40,41] See **Fig. 9** for other systemic involvement signs and symptoms.

Differential Diagnosis

- The manifestation of another collagen vascular disease
- Mixed connective tissue disease
- Heliotrope rash of dermatomyositis (DM)
- Seborrheic dermatitis
- Rosacea

Diagnosis

Laboratory tests aid in the diagnosis of suspected cutaneous lupus, along with the history and physical examination. Even in those without suspected systemic involvement, laboratory tests should still be done because of the possibility of development of systemic disease later. These tests include the following:

- CBC
- ESR and CRP

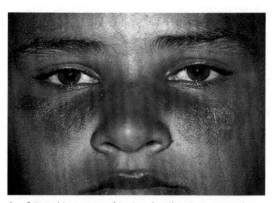

Fig. 8. Butterfly rash of SLE. (*Courtesy of* Freire da Silva S. Dermatology Atlas. Available at: http://www.atlasdermatologico.com.br/index.jsf. Accessed April 25, 2015.)

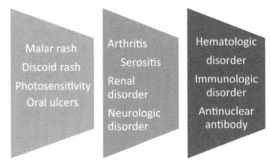

Fig. 9. Systemic manifestations (one needs 4 of 11 manifestations to be diagnosed with SLE).

- ANA
- Anti-dsDNA and anti-Smith antibodies
- Anti-Ro and anti-La autoantibodies
- Anti-ribonucleoprotein
- Urinary analysis (UA)
- Complement values of C3 and C4
- Anti-phospholipid antibodies
- Venereal disease research laboratory test (VDRL)

Skin biopsy shows vacuolar degeneration of the basal cell layer and perivascular lymphocytic infiltrate. With immunofluorescence, complement deposits can be seen along the dermal-epidermal junction. Speckled IgG deposits may also be observed in basal cell cytoplasm associated with Ro/La antibodies. Skin biopsy has now largely been replaced by serologic testing.[38]

Treatment

Treatment should be coordinated with Rheumatology and varies from patient to patient. Treatment can change with time depending on whether active flares are present. Readdressing treatment and potential treatment changes are needed on a frequent basis. Treatment also depends on the presence of systemic symptoms as opposed to pure cutaneous symptoms. Main treatments include the following:

- Sun avoidance, sunscreen use, layered/protective clothing
- Topical steroids
  - Triamcinolone and fluinonide cream
- Hydroxychloroquine
- Oral steroids if resistant to topical. Oral steroids have many side effects with long-term use (**Fig. 10**)
- Alternatives for severe skin manifestations and those who are resistant
  - Azathioprine, MTX, thalidomide, isoretinoin, and dapsone

Prognosis

Prognosis is variable. The 5-year survival rate is greater than 90%; the 10-year survival rate is 80%. There is a worse prognosis if systemic symptoms are present, particularly nephritis.[38,41] There is a worse prognosis in men than in women. The most common causes of death are renal disease, sepsis, and iatrogenic infection secondary to immunosuppression.[40,42]

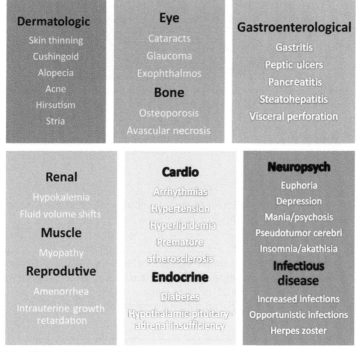

Fig. 10. Side effects of oral steroids.

DISCOID LUPUS ERYTHEMATOUS
Definition

Discoid lupus erythematosus is a different type of rash that can occur in lupus. It is known for its tendency to cause scarring and involvement of the hair follicles and may be part of the syndrome of systemic lupus. However, often, it presents purely as skin manifestations.

Epidemiology

This condition affects young and old individuals with an incidence of 2 per 1000.[41]

Clinical Presentation

The rash may be slightly pruritic with positive relation to sun exposure/exacerbation. Patients may have history of systemic disease complaints but often are asymptomatic.

The lesions are sharply demarcated plaques, erythematous, pruritic, and round disks. They can occur anywhere but favor the face and scalp. Often a scale that penetrates into the hair follicles can be appreciated. When this scale is removed, carpet tracks, or small spiny projections of keratinous plugs, may be present. Atrophy occurs in both the dermis and epidermis, which is not seen in systemic lupus. Hypopigmentation, hyperpigmentation, and hypertrophic changes can be seen and can cause disfigurement. Lesions on the scalp may be present, which is associated with scarring alopecia (**Fig. 11**).

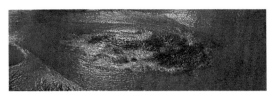

Fig. 11. Discoid lupus. (*Courtesy of* Freire da Silva S. Dermatology Atlas. Available at: http://www.atlasdermatologico.com.br/index.jsf. Accessed April 25, 2015.)

Differential Diagnosis

- Psoriasis
- LP
- SLE

Key point: Hyperkeratosis, follicular plugging, vacuolar degeneration, scarring, and atrophic plaques limited to skin finding is probable discoid lupus.

Diagnosis

Diagnosis is made by performing similar laboratory tests as seen in systemic SLE, as well as a complete history and physical examination. It is rare to have anti-dsDNA in discoid lupus, an ESR more than 30, or false-positive VDRL/syphilis. Issues with anemia are also less common, compared with the prevalence in SLE.[38,40,41]

Treatment

Treatment should be coordinated with Dermatology and Rheumatology and is similar to SLE treatment. Topical steroids are often enough to treat fully. Dermatology may also use intralesional steroid injections.

Prognosis

Prognosis is good. The disease is often controllable, with remission occurring on its own in 50% of the cases.[42] Scarring and postinflammatory hyperpigmentation are often a concern. Permanent alopecia of the scalp may also occur. The risk of developing SLE is low (5%–10%).[42]

HELIOTROPE RASH AND GOTTRON PAPULES OF DERMATOMYOSITIS
Definition

DM is an autoimmune inflammatory muscle disease that can be associated with malignancy. The clinical picture varies considerably, but proximal muscle weakness is the most prevalent presenting manifestation. About 40% of patients present with muscle weakness as the initial finding.[38,43]

Other common presentations are arthralgia, dysphagia, myocardial inflammation, and respiratory muscle weakness, which can lead to interstitial pneumonitis and aspiration pneumonia. A compatible muscle biopsy and elevated creatine phosphokinase (CPK) and aldolase levels are other major criteria.

The dermatologic manifestations that are pathognomonic for DM are the heliotrope rash and Gottron papules.

Epidemiology

The disease is rare, occurring only in 10 in 1 million. However, this number does not reflect childhood cases, elderly cases, overlap cases, and cases that do not involve muscles.[38,43]

Key point: In patients with onset more than age 55 years, associated malignancy should be ruled out.

Clinical Presentation

In DM, the main clinical presentation is myositis/muscle inflammation, skin manifestations, or both. Patients complain of difficulty rising from a chair, combing one's hair, climbing stairs or swallowing/choking on food, which can lead to possible recurrent pneumonia. Other complaints include chest pain, skin rash/lesions, periorbital edema/swelling of the eyelids, flushing, scaling, and desquamation. The most common area of change is the eyelids, but skin manifestation may involve the entire face, scalp, upper arms, and chest. The rash does not itch and is not painful.

Key point: The heliotrope rash (violet rash) is considered classic. Violet/purple coloration is seen, which may be observed around the eyelids (**Fig. 12**).

Gottron papules is the other skin manifestation that is considered pathognomonic for DM. They are round, violet, smooth, small (<1 cm), flat papules seen over bony prominences. They are particularly located over the knuckles and along the side of the fingers (**Fig. 13**). They can also be located at the nape of the neck, shoulders, and elbows. Approximately 60% to 80% of patients with DM at one point have Gottron papules.[38,43]

Other skin manifestations of DM include the following:

- Periungual erythema: irregular red streaks at the nail fold; thick cuticles; rough, hyperkeratotic, moth-eaten appearance of the nails
- Telangiectasia: small dilated blood vessels near the surface of the skin and mucous membranes, similar to what is seen in SLE, and scleroderma (Sc)
- Poikiloderma: occurs late in the course of the disease and has a characteristic pattern of finely mottled white areas with areas of hypopigmentation/hyperpigmentation, telangiectasia, and atrophy. This condition can also be seen in SLE, Sc, and mycosis fungoides.[42]

Differential Diagnosis

- Lupus
- Mixed connective tissue disease
- Steroid myopathy
- Trichinosis
- Toxoplasmosis
- Lyme disease

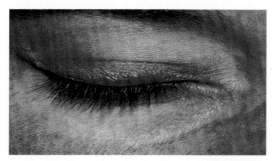

Fig. 12. Heliotrope rash. (*Courtesy of* Freire da Silva S. Dermatology Atlas. Available at: http://www.atlasdermatologico.com.br/index.jsf. Accessed April 25, 2015.)

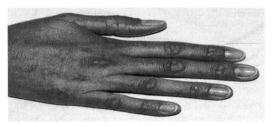

Fig. 13. Gottron papules. (*Courtesy of* Freire da Silva S. Dermatology Atlas. Available at: http://www.atlasdermatologico.com.br/index.jsf. Accessed April 25, 2015.)

- Muscular dystrophy
- Amyotrophic lateral sclerosis

Diagnosis

Diagnosis is made with a complete history and physical examination. Laboratory tests aid in the diagnosis of suspected DM or polymyositis and include the following:

- ANA
- ESR, CRP
- SS-A, SS-B (Ro/LA) antibodies
- Anti-KU
  - Associated with overlap syndrome of SLE/Sc/myositis
  - Anti-ribonucleoprotein (RNP) mixed connective tissue disease[39,41,44]
- Muscle enzymes
  - Alanine aminotransferase, aspartate aminotransferase, and lactate dehydrogenase
  - 24-hour urine creatinine
  - Aldolase and CPK

Not all of these laboratory test values need to be elevated, and they can change over time, improving or worsening. They may also be used to measure disease activity. CPK is often used to monitor disease activity.

- Muscle biopsy/electromyography
  - Several biopsies may need to be taken. Biopsy should be taken from a proximal muscle. Biopsy of areas that have had recent steroid injection should be avoided.
- MRI can be used to identify affected areas in need of biopsy.
- Key point: Evaluation should be done for possible malignancy in patients older than 55 years.
  - Lung, ovary, pancreas, stomach, colon, lymphomas, and ear-nose-throat cancers in particular

Treatment

Treatment should be coordinated with Dermatology and Rheumatology.

As with most autoimmune diseases, steroids are the number one treatment. Oral steroids are often given for DM. Adjuvant therapy may be required in those who do not respond to steroids alone. Azathioprine and MTX are most often used as adjuvants. For the cutaneous manifestation alone, topical steroids are used, as well as immunomodulators, which include tacrolimus ointment and pimecrolimus creams. Other treatments include sunscreens, sun avoidance, and hydroxychloroquine sulfate.

Key point: Hydroxychloroquine sulfate does not help with muscle disease. Annual examinations are needed for hydroxychloroquine sulfate use because of potential eye changes with its use.

MTX, mycophenolate mofetil, azathioprine, cyclophosphamide, cholorambucil, and cyclosporine may be used in the setting of systemic manifestation and resistant disease. MTX is the first-line adjuvant therapy. Side effects, however, must be monitored closely. Side effects include stomatitis, GI distress, pneumonitis, headache, alopecia, itching, fever, neutropenia, liver fibrosis, and cirrhosis.

When a patient is administered MTX, a liver biopsy may be needed before treatment in at-risk patients. Folate supplements should be taken with MTX. Liver function test and CBC should be monitored periodically. Woman of childbearing age should be given oral contraceptives as MTX is teratogenic. There is an increased risk of non-Hodgkin lymphoma and other lymphomas with MTX.

Other treatment includes physical therapy to prevent atrophy and contractures. Once pain has decreased, aggressive programs should be started to prevent loss of muscle mass. Lastly, patients with dysphagia due to muscle weakness should follow aspiration precautions.

Prognosis

Prognosis is poor/guarded. The prognosis in DM is worse in those with dysphagia, pulmonary disease, and malignancy. Prognosis is improved in those without significant elevations in CPK levels or who have a strong response to oral steroids alone. The 8-year survival rate with treatment is 70% to 80%.[43,44]

SKIN SCLEROSIS AND RAYNAUD PHENOMENON OF SCLERODERMA
Definition

Sc is an autoimmune multisystem disorder that involves inflammation of the skin; sclerosis means a hardening of the tissue/skin, blood vessels, and internal organs. The lungs, heart, and GI tract are particularly affected. Skin hardening occurs because of an excess of collagen fibers.

Sc can present in 2 different forms. The limited form involves skin changes of the hands, face, feet, and forearms only (this includes CREST syndrome) and accounts for about 65% of cases. The autoantibody usually associated with this form is anti-centrometric antibody.[38,45]

The diffuse form has a more rapid onset involving the same areas, plus the trunk, synovitis, tendons, and most importantly, internal organs. The prognosis for this form is much worse. The autoantibody associated with this form is Scl-70/anti-topoisomerase I.[38,45]

As the name suggests, the main dermatologic manifestation is hardening of the skin. Raynaud phenomenon (vasoconstriction of vessels in the digits), sclerodactyly, hair loss, nail changes, and telangiectasias may also be seen.

Epidemiology

The prevalence of Sc is 20 cases per 1 million in the United States. Average age of onset is 30 to 40 years. Women are 4 times more likely to be affected.[42,45]

Clinical Presentation

The main presentation is sclerosis of the skin (hardening of the skin) (**Fig. 14**). Ninety-eight percent of patients present with skin that looks waxy, shiny, stretched, and hard/tightly bound down.[45] The normal wrinkle lines are distorted or absent, making people appear younger than chronologic age. They appear to have a masklike facies with thin

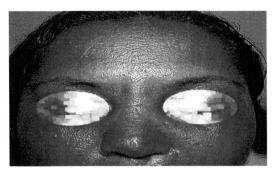

Fig. 14. Sclerosis. (*Courtesy of* Freire da Silva S. Dermatology Atlas. Available at: http://www. atlasdermatologico.com.br/index.jsf. Accessed April 25, 2015.)

lips and beaklike nose. This skin sclerosis can eventually lead to contractures and a leatherlike appearance of the skin.

The other main manifestation of Sc is Raynaud disease, which is present 90% of the time.[42] Raynaud disease causes areas of the body, particularly fingers and toes, to feel numb and cold in response to cold temperatures or stress; this is due to vasoconstriction of the vessels, which can lead to ischemia, painful ulcerations, and even gangrene. There is a classic triphasic color change from pale to cyanosis to rubor (**Fig. 15**).

A late manifestation in Sc is sclerodactyly, which is atrophy of the underlying soft tissues and bony reabsorption leading to shortening of the fingers. Other presentations in Sc are loss of sweat glands, loss of hair over distal extremities, hyperpigmentation, and oral ulcers. See **Fig. 16** for other systemic manifestations seen in Sc.

CREST SYNDROME

CREST syndrome is a variant of the limited form of Sc. The acronym stands for

- Calcinosis cutis
- Raynaud disease
- Esophageal dysfunction

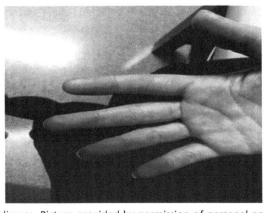

Fig. 15. Raynaud disease. Picture provided by permission of personal patient.

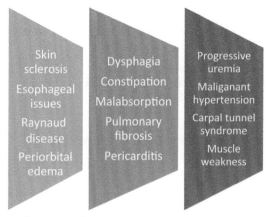

Fig. 16. Systemic manifestations of Sc.

- Sclerodactyly
- Telangiectasia

Calcinosis cutis is a condition in which there are calcium deposits in the skin (**Fig. 17**), which can be seen on radiographs.

The main esophageal dysfunction complaints are reflux, slowed peristalsis, dysphagia, and constipation. Telangiectasias are often macular and located on the face and trunk and sometimes on the scalp. They are small dilated blood vessels near the surface of the skin.

Differential Diagnosis

- Mixed connective tissue disease
- Eosinophilic fasciitis
- Morphea
- Porphyria cutanea tarda
- Lichen sclerosis
- Polyvinyl chloride exposure
- Drugs such as β-blockers, bleomycin, or botulinum toxin

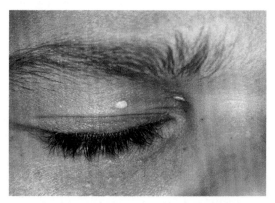

Fig. 17. Calcinosis cutis. (*Courtesy of* Freire da Silva S. Dermatology Atlas. Available at: http://www.atlasdermatologico.com.br/index.jsf. Accessed April 25, 2015.)

Diagnosis

History and physical examination are key. Laboratory evaluation includes the following:

- ANA, CBC, UA, renal function test
- Chest radiography and pulmonary function test
- Autoantibodies SS-A/SS-B, Smith
- Anti-nRNP
- Barium swallow
- Annual echocardiography for heart disease screening
- Scl-70, anti-centromere
- Deep skin biopsy
- Nailfold microscopy

Treatment

Treatment of systemic Sc can be difficult, often with poor response to medications. Treatment is supportive, not curative. Because Sc presents in so many ways, treatment often must be tailored and changed periodically based on the patient's symptoms and course of disease. Treatment should involve management with Rheumatology and Dermatology.

For skin manifestations alone, topical and interlesional steroids are often used. Oral steroids may be used for more systemic symptoms and resistant diseases.

Key point: High-dose steroids should be avoided to avoid triggering Sc renal crisis.

D-Penicillamine may also be used as treatment. It prevents cross-linking of collagen fibers, but treatment should be followed up with monthly CBCs and UA. Research has not confirmed its efficacy.

Immunosuppressive argents, primarily MTX and mycophenolate, are also used but have many side effects discussed earlier. Cyclophosphamide is usually reserved for refractory cases, patients with pulmonary complications or severe rapidly progressing skin changes. For patients with advanced localized skin lesions photochemotherapy (Psoraten Ultraviolet A Therapy) may be helpful.

Raynaud phenomenon can stand alone but is often seen in Sc. It has its own treatment. The initial treatment is preventing exposure to cold, limiting stress, and dressing the entire body warmly. The use of gloves and hand warmers is effective. Smoking cessation is essential. Patient should avoid decongestants, amphetamines, attention-deficit disorder medications, and migraine medications. Pharmacotherapy involves calcium channel blockers such as nifedipine or amlodipine. For resistant Raynaud disease, sildenafil, topical nitrates, losartan, prazosin, fluoxetine, and botulinum toxin can be used.[46]

Prognosis

Systemic Sc has a poor prognosis. Death from systemic involvement is not uncommon.

The 5-year survival rate is estimated at 40% to 80%, depending mostly on the extent of visceral organ involvement.[45] Renal diseases with malignant hypertension are the leading cause of death, followed by cardiac disease and pulmonary complications such as fibrosis. Infections from steroid treatment/immune modulators, leading to opportunistic infections, can lead to sepsis and severe complications. Cutaneous manifestation alone and limited Sc often have a much better prognosis, with the disease burning itself out, which can take years. However, skin may never fully return to normal, with hyperpigmentation/hypopigmentation remaining.[38,45]

MORPHEA

Definition

Morphea is a localized well-circumscribed oval or linear cutaneous form of sclerosis. It begins spontaneously and involves thickening of the skin like Sc, but is unrelated to systemic Sc and CREST syndrome. Violet borders and later ivory skin changes are characteristic of the disease.

Epidemiology

Morphea is more common in women by about 3-fold. However, linear morphea affects both men and women equally. It tends to occur after the age of 30 years.[42]

Clinical Presentation

In morphea, patients lack systemic symptoms. Unlike in Sc, the areas start originally as well-circumscribed violet lesions, round, oval, or linear (**Fig. 18**). Over months to years, the lesions progress to the thick/firm skin appearance of that of Sc. Then, they change to ivory color but maintain their violet border, called the lilac ring. Although it may take 1 to 25 years, the lesion may resolve completely. The underlying tissues and muscles are not usually involved.[41,42] Lesions may also involve the tongue, nails, and scalp. Lesions can cross the joint lines and cause contractures that can be disabling.

Differential Diagnosis

- Sc
- Acrodermatitis atrophicans
- Lichen sclerosis
- Lyme disease

Diagnosis

In addition to history and physical examination, laboratory evaluation includes the following:

- Lyme titers
- ANA, anti-DNA, anti-histone antibodies
- Biopsy
  - Inflammatory cells in the dermis and subcutaneous tissues, eosinophils, and a loss of rete ridges
  - Later in the disease, thickening of the dermis with fibroblast and dense collagen

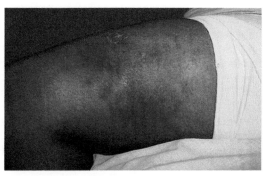

Fig. 18. Morphea. (*Courtesy of* Freire da Silva S. Dermatology Atlas. Available at: http://www. atlasdermatologico.com.br/index.jsf. Accessed April 25, 2015.)

Treatment/Prognosis

Prognosis is excellent. There is no effective treatment for morphea. Low-dose, limited treatments with oral and topical steroids may be helpful but have limited proven efficacy. Given the thickness of most lesions, penetration of topical steroids can be difficult. For linear morphea and juvenile morphea, physical therapy is started to prevent contractures from forming. Asymptomatic lesions are often and should be left alone.[42]

SUMMARY

Certain dermatologic conditions can be associated with systemic illness. Patients may present initially with a dermatologic complaint. Therefore, the primary care physician should be familiar with the dermatologic sequela of systemic diseases. Initial evaluation almost always involves various laboratory studies. Treatment is specific to the particular underlying diagnosis. It can include surveillance with clinical evaluations and laboratory monitoring, pharmacotherapy with topical or oral medications such as steroids or immune modulators, and directed treatment of the underlying systemic condition. Consultation with various subspecialists, such as Dermatology, Rheumatology, and Gastroenterology, may be warranted for particular conditions that require further management.

REFERENCES

1. Aseni P, Di Sandro S, Mihaylov P, et al. Atypical presentation of pyoderma gangrenosum complicating ulcerative colitis: rapid disappearance with methylprednisolone. World J Gastroenterol 2008;14(35):5471–3.
2. Brooklyn J, Dunnill G, Probert C. Diagnosis and treatment of pyoderma gangrenosa. BMJ 2006;33(7560):181–4.
3. Wollina U. Pyoderma gangrenosum–a review. Orphanet J Rare Dis 2007;2:19.
4. Ruocco E, Sangiuliano S, Gravina AG, et al. Pyoderma gangrenosum: an updated review. J Eur Acad Dermatol Venereol 2009;23:1008.
5. Schadt C, Jeffery C, Ofori A. Pyoderma gangrenosum: pathologenesis, clinical features and diagnosis. Up to Date; 2014.
6. Marks J, Miller J. Principles of dermatology. Philadelphia: Elsevier Inc; 2006.
7. Schwartz RA, Nervi SJ. Erythema nodosum: a sign of systemic disease. Am Fam Physician 2007;75(5):695–700.
8. Marshal JK, Irvine EJ. Successful therapy of refractory erythema nodosum associated with Crohn's disease using potassium iodide. Can J Gastroenterol 1997; 11:501–2.
9. Requena L, Yus ES. Erythema nodosum. Dermatol Clin 2008;4:425–38.
10. Tremane WJ. Treatment of erythema nodosum, apthous stomatitis and pyoderma gangrenosum in patients with IBD. Inflamm Bowel Dis 1998;4:68–9.
11. Gilchrist H, Patterson JW. Erythema nodosum and erythema induratum (nodular vasculitis): diagnosis and management. Dermatol Ther 2010;4:320–7.
12. Preeti L, Magesh KT, Rajkumar K, et al. Recurrent aphthous stomatitis. J Oral Maxillofac Pathol 2011;15:252–6.
13. Casiglia J, Mirowski G, Nebesio C, et al. Apthous stomatitis. Medscape; 2014.
14. Bolotin D, Petronic-Rosic V. Dermatitis herpetiformis: part I. Epidemiology, pathogenesis and clinical presentation. J Am Acad Dermatol 2011;64(6):1017–24.
15. Dieterich W, Laag E, Bruckner-Tuderman L, et al. Antibodies to tissue transglutaminase as serologic markers in patients with dermatitis herpetiformis. J Invest Dermatol 1999;113(1):133.

16. Rose C, Armbruster FP, Ruppert J, et al. Autoantibodies against epidermal transglutaminase are a sensitive diagnostic marker in patients with dermatitis herpetiformis on a normal or gluten-free diet. J Am Acad Dermatol 2009; 61(1):39–43.

17. Egan CA, O'Loughlin S, Gormally S, et al. Dermatitis herpetiformis: a review of fifty-four patients. Ir J Med Sci 1997;166:241.

18. Alonso-Llamazares J, Gibson LE, Rogers RS 3rd. Clinical, pathologic, and immunopathologic features of dermatitis herpetiformis: review of the Mayo Clinic experience. Int J Dermatol 2007;46(9):910–9.

19. Zone JJ, Meyer LJ, Petersen MJ. Deposition of granular IgA relative to clinical lesions in dermatitis herpetiformis. Arch Dermatol 1996;132(8):912–8.

20. Fry L, Leonard JN, Swain F, et al. Long term follow-up of dermatitis herpetiformis with and without dietary gluten withdrawal. Br J Dermatol 1982;107(6):631–40.

21. Karpati S. Dermatitis Herpetiformis. Clin Dermatol 2012;30(1):56–9.

22. Lehman JS, Tollefson MM, Gibson LE. Lichen planus. Int J Dermatol 2009;48:682.

23. Usatine RP, Tinitigan M. Diagnosis and treatment of lichen planus. Am Fam Physician 2011;84(1):53–60.

24. Pandhi D, Singal A, Bhattacharya SN. Lichen planus in childhood: a series of 316 patients. Pediatr Dermatol 2014;31:59.

25. Başak PY, Başak K. Generalized lichen planus in childhood: is dapsone an effective treatment modality? Turk J Pediatr 2002;44:346.

26. Lallas A, Kyrgidis A, Tzellos TG, et al. Accuracy of dermoscopic criteria for the diagnosis of psoriasis, dermatitis, lichen planus and pityriasis rosea. Br J Dermatol 2012;166:1198.

27. Bauzá A, España A, Gil P, et al. Successful treatment of lichen planus with sulfasalazine in 20 patients. Int J Dermatol 2005;44:158.

28. Büyük AY, Kavala M. Oral metronidazole treatment of lichen planus. J Am Acad Dermatol 2000;43:260.

29. Cribier B, Frances C, Chosidow O. Treatment of lichen planus. An evidence-based medicine analysis of efficacy. Arch Dermatol 1998;134:1521.

30. Frieling U, Bonsmann G, Schwarz T, et al. Treatment of severe lichen planus with mycophenolate mofetil. J Am Acad Dermatol 2003;49:1063.

31. Laurberg G, Geiger JM, Hjorth N, et al. Treatment of lichen planus with acitretin. A double-blind, placebo-controlled study in 65 patients. J Am Acad Dermatol 1991; 24:434.

32. Nousari HC, Goyal S, Anhalt GJ. Successful treatment of resistant hypertrophic and bullous lichen planus with mycophenolate mofetil. Arch Dermatol 1999; 135:1420.

33. Rasi A, Behzadi AH, Davoudi S, et al. Efficacy of oral metronidazole in treatment of cutaneous and mucosal lichen planus. J Drugs Dermatol 2010;9:1186.

34. Sehgal VN, Abraham GJ, Malik GB. Griseofulvin therapy in lichen planus. A double-blind controlled trial. Br J Dermatol 1972;87:383.

35. Lu SY, Chen WJ, Eng HL. Dramatic response to levamisole and low dose prednisolone in 23 patients with oral lichen planus: a 6-year prospective follow-up study. Oral Surg Oral Med Oral Pathol Oral Radiol Endod 1995;80(6):705–9.

36. Tai HW, Se YP, Bo SK, et al. Levamisole monotherapy for oral lichen planus. Ann Dermatol 2009;21(3):250–4.

37. Carbone M, Arduino PG, Carrozzo M, et al. Course of oral lichen planus: a retrospective study of 808 northern Italian patients. Oral Dis 2009;15:235.

38. Habif T. Clinical dermatology, a color guide to diagnosis and therapy. 5th edition. Honover (Germany): Mosby Elsevier; 2010.

39. Hertl M. Autoimmune diseases of the skin, pathogenesis, diagnosis, management. 2nd edition. New York: Springer Wien; 2005.
40. Schur P, Hahn B. Epidemiology and pathogenesis of systemic lupus erythematosus. UpToDate; 2014. Web: December 18, 2014.
41. Marks J, Miller J. Looking Bill and Marks' principles of dermatology. 4th edition. Philadelphia: Saunders Elsvier; 2006.
42. Wolff K, Johnson R, Saavedra A. Fitzpatricks' color atlas and synopsis of clinical dermatology. 7th edition. New York: McGraw Hill; 2013.
43. Vleugels RA. Initial management of cutaneous dermatomyositis. UpToDate; 2014. Web: January 18, 2014.
44. Koopman W, Boulware D, Heudebent G. Clinical primer of rheumatology. 1st edition. Philidephia: LWW; 2003.
45. Denton C. Overview of the treatment and prognosis of systemic sclerosis (scleroderma) in adults. UpToDate; 2014. Web: January 2, 2015.
46. Wisley F. Initial treatment of the raynaud phenomenon. UpToDate; 2014. Web: January 18, 2015.

Pressure and Friction Injuries in Primary Care

Shawn Phillips, MD, MSPT[a,b,c,*], Elizabeth Seiverling, MD[d],
Matthew Silvis, MD[a,b,c]

KEYWORDS

- Pressure injury • Friction injury • Skin breakdown • Athletes • Ulcer • Intertrigo

KEY POINTS

- Pressure and friction injuries are common throughout the lifespan.
- A detailed history of the onset and progression of friction and pressure injuries is key to aiding clinicians in determining the underlying mechanism behind the development of the injury.
- Modifying or removing the forces that are creating pressure or friction is the key to both prevention and healing of these injuries.
- Proper care of pressure and friction injuries to the skin is important to prevent the development of infection.
- Patient education on positioning and ergonomics can help to prevent recurrence of pressure and friction injuries.

INTRODUCTION

Injuries to the skin caused by pressure or friction are common throughout the lifespan. Dermatologic problems are consistently among the most common reasons patients see a primary care provider.[1,2] In healthy individuals, pressure and friction injuries tend to occur as a result of repetitive stress leading to pain and skin breakdown. Breakdown of the natural barrier provided by the integument can lead to infection. For individuals with altered sensation or mobility limitations, these injuries are potentially serious and should be recognized and treated quickly. Skin injury attributed to prolonged pressure includes minor problems such as corns and talon noir, as well

[a] Department of Family and Community Medicine, 500 University Drive, H154, Hershey, PA 17033, USA; [b] Department of Orthopedics and Rehabilitation, 500 University Drive, Hershey, PA 17033, USA; [c] Penn State Primary Care Sports Medicine Fellowship, Department of Family and Community Medicine, Penn State Milton S. Hershey Medical Center, 500 University Drive, H154, Hershey, PA 17033, USA; [d] Department of Dermatology, Penn State Hershey Dermatology, 500 University Drive, UPC 1, Suite 100, Hershey, PA 17033, USA
* Corresponding author. Department of Family and Community Medicine, 500 University Drive, H154, Hershey, PA 17033.
E-mail address: sphillips6@hmc.psu.edu

Prim Care Clin Office Pract 42 (2015) 631–644
http://dx.doi.org/10.1016/j.pop.2015.07.002
0095-4543/15/$ – see front matter © 2015 Elsevier Inc. All rights reserved.
primarycare.theclinics.com

as pressure ulcers, which carry more significant morbidity. Injuries to the skin caused by friction include chafing and intertrigo, abrasions, blisters, and acne mechanica (also called frictional folliculitis). This article discusses the diagnosis and management of common pressure and friction injuries, which are listed in **Table 1**.

PRESSURE INJURY
Pressure Ulcer

History
Pressure ulcer is a common problem in the United States and around the world. Pressure ulcers disproportionally affect the elderly and infirm.[3] They are common in hospital and nursing home settings and are often encountered by primary care providers who care for patients in these environments or see them in the office or a home visit after discharge. Risk factors for developing pressure ulcers include increased age, immobility, neurologic impairment (as in spinal cord injury or stroke), compromise to blood flow (such as in diabetes mellitus with neuropathy), poor nutritional status, and incontinence. The Braden Scale is commonly used in the inpatient setting to identify patients who are at higher risk for pressure ulcer in an effort to prevent such injuries.[3–5] Prevention of ulcers by determining risk is an area of ongoing study.[6]

Patients at high risk for the development of a pressure ulcer should be evaluated regularly during primary care encounters with a goal of prevention or early identification. **Table 2** lists risk factors for development of pressure ulcer.

Examination
Evaluation for pressure ulcer begins with examination of skin in high-risk areas, including bony prominences of the low back/sacrum, greater trochanters, knees, malleoli, plantar surfaces, shoulders, scapulae, and occiput.[4,5] When a pressure ulcer is identified it is classified into one of the stages listed in **Table 3**. Stages I to IV are illustrated in **Fig. 1**.

For patients who are bedbound, high-risk areas include the sacrum, scapulae, and greater trochanters. For spinal cord–injured patients who use a wheelchair for locomotion, the ischial region is commonly affected. Patients with lower limb neuropathy, especially patients with diabetes, are at risk for heel and plantar surface ulcers. Understanding a patient's baseline activity level and mobility limitations helps guide examination.

Poor nutritional status is a risk factor for the development of pressure ulcers. The National Pressure Ulcer Advisory Panel recommends evaluation of nutritional status in the primary prevention of pressure ulcers.[4,7] Screening questionnaires such as the Mini Nutritional Assessment Questionnaire have been developed to help primary care providers screen for nutritional deficiencies in elderly patients.[8,9] For individuals at risk of skin breakdown, a larger percentage of daily intake should come from

Table 1	
Pressure and friction injuries	
Pressure	**Friction**
Pressure ulcer	Intertrigo
Corns and calluses	Blisters
Talon noir (black heel)	Abrasions
Subungual hematoma	Acne mechanica

Table 2 Risk factors for pressure ulcer disease	
Age	Increased age leads to Increased risk of skin breakdown
Nutritional status	Low body mass (BMI <18.5) Extremely obese (BMI >40) Inadequate protein
Activity and mobility level	Bedbound or wheelchair-bound individuals are at high risk for breakdown over bony prominences. Patients who transfer by sliding between surfaces are at risk for friction injury
Limited sensation	Areas of skin with decreased sensation caused by spinal cord injury or neuropathy are at high risk for skin breakdown
Oxygen status	Patients with poor baseline oxygenation, such as in CHF and COPD, especially those requiring oxygen, are at higher risk for breakdown because of poor oxygen perfusion of skin
Baseline skin condition	Individuals with current or previous skin breakdown are at high risk for further pressure ulceration
Incontinence	Bowel or bladder incontinence increases risk of skin irritation and breakdown

Abbreviations: BMI, body mass index; CHF, congestive heart failure; COPD, chronic obstructive pulmonary disease.
Adapted from National Pressure Ulcer Advisory Panel and European Pressure Ulcer Advisory Panel. Prevention and treatment of pressure ulcer: clinical practice guideline. Washington, DC: National Pressure Ulcer Advisory Panel; 2009.

sources high in protein.[10,11] Zinc, vitamin C, and arginine are sometimes supplemented in patients with pressure ulcers. However, studies have not shown consistent in vivo wound healing benefit in patients taking greater than the recommended daily intake of these supplements.[10,12]

Physical examination of any pressure ulcer should include measurements of length, width, and depth as well as the degree of tissue loss, location of the wound, and the character of the wound, including the presence or absence of exudate, and, if present, the type and amount.[4] Once these characteristics are known, the wound can be staged (see Table 3).

Table 3 Stages of pressure ulcer	
Stage	Description
Stage I	Nonblanchable area of redness of intact skin
Stage II	Partial-thickness skin loss or blister. Presentations may include a shallow erosion or ulceration, an intact or flaccid bulla
Stage III	Full-thickness skin loss with adipose tissue visible. Bone, muscle, and tendon are not exposed. May be some slough
Stage IV	Full-thickness injury with bone, muscle, or tendon visible
Unstageable	Full-thickness tissue loss with unknown depth because the wound is obscured by slough or eschar. Once debrided, stage can be assigned
Suspected deep tissue injury	Localized purple or dark red area of discolored but intact skin. Can also be a blister filled with blood. Results from underlying tissue damage caused by pressure or shear forces

Adapted from Bluestein D, Javaheri A. Pressure ulcers: prevention, evaluation, and management. Am Fam Physician 2008;78(10):1186–94.

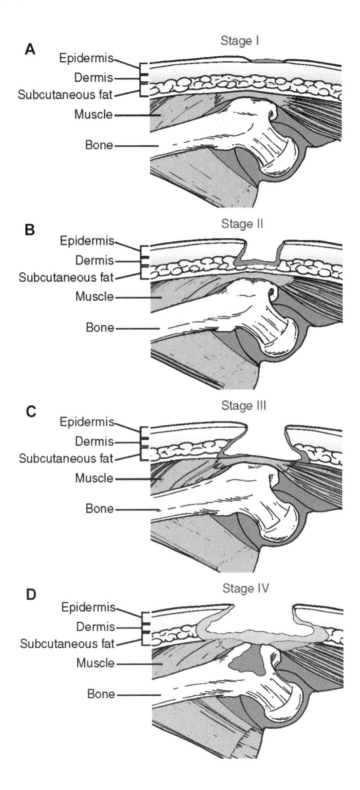

Treatment

Treatment of pressure ulcer is best accomplished with the help of a multidisciplinary team that is experienced in wound care. The main goals of treatment are to remove any necrotic tissue, relieve or avoid pressure on the injured area, and prevent infection. There are multiple wound dressings that may be used to achieve these goals. Use of dressing is determined by several factors, including the depth of the wound and the quality and quantity of exudate. **Table 4** lists common dressings and their respective indications.

Along with the dressings described, treatment with a topical or systemic antibiotic should be initiated in any wound with cellulitis and considered for wounds that are not showing improvement within 2 weeks of treatment. Necrotic wounds may be a nidus of infection and should be treated with some type of debridement, one exception being heel ulcers that are covered with necrotic tissue but appear stable and are not infected, which do not need to be debrided.[13] Sharp debridement either at the bedside or, in more extensive cases, in the operating room is quick and effective. The goal of debridement is to remove dead tissue and allow healthy granulation tissue to proliferate. The remaining wound is then treated with one of the dressings listed in **Table 4**.

The mainstay of treatment of pressure ulcers is modification of forces that can contribute to breakdown. For bedbound patients, use of mattresses that distribute forces throughout the body and away from bony prominences is paramount. Gel or static air mattresses can reduce pressures for patients who are mobile. These mattresses are adequate for those patients who are able to adhere to a turning schedule or are actively mobile while in bed. For those patients who are less mobile, an air flow mattress that is constantly changing the pressure under the patient is preferred. Choice of mattress is determined by a multitude of factors, including mobility of the patient, stage of the wound, and cost of the mattress.

Selection of seating surface is also important in the healing of sacral and ischial pressure wounds. Position of the seat and seat back alter pressure on the sacral and ischial regions.[14] Chairs may be custom fitted to the patient to minimize pressure and allow healing. Chairs with adjustable backs allow position changes in order to relieve pressure. A variety of seat cushions are available, ranging from static foam and gel surfaces to cushions with multiple air-filled bladders to distribute force. Referral to physical or occupational therapists who are experienced in wheelchair fitting and positioning can ensure that patient mobility is maximized and the risk of worsening pressure sores is minimized.

Similarly, patients with foot ulcers should have a thorough evaluation of their footwear. Diabetic patients are at particularly high risk for plantar surface ulcerations because of a combination of decreased sensation caused by neuropathy and decreased vascular flow. Footwear that has a wide toe box and well-distributed plantar forces is important in the prevention and healing of diabetic ulcers.[13,15]

Treatment of pressure sores should also include nutritional education. Although evidence is limited, there is little doubt that adequate nutrition is important in the healing process. Daily recommended protein intake is 1.5 to 2.0 g/kg/d.[7] Increased caloric intake through liquid supplementation can be helpful in the elderly with decreased

Fig. 1. (*A*) Stage I pressure ulcer showing nonblanchable intact dermis. (*B*) Stage II ulcer with partial-thickness skin loss into the dermis. (*C*) Stage III ulcer with full-thickness skin loss through the dermis with visible adipose. (*D*) Stage IV ulcer with full-thickness injury with exposure of muscle and bone. (*From* Buck CJ. Step-by-step medical coding. New York: Elsevier Saunders; 2011; with permission.)

Table 4	
Dressings used in the care of pressure ulcers	
Dressing Type	**Indication**
Transparent gel	Adhesive semipermeable barrier. Used for stage 1 and 2 wounds. Maintains moisture, decreases risk of infection
Hydrogel	Water-based or glycerin-based gel dressing. May be impregnated into gauze. Reduces pain. Hydration to wound bed. Autodebridement. Can pack the wound. Helpful in infections
Alginate	Pads derived from seaweed. Very absorbent. Can be used on stage II, III, or IV wounds with heavy exudate
Foam	Pads or sheets. Primary or secondary dressing for stage II–IV wounds. Can be used for moderate to severe exudate
Hydrocolloid	Occlusive or semiocclusive dressing. Provides barrier to infection. Autodebridement

Adapted from Hess CT. Wound care. 4th edition. Springhouse (PA): Springhouse; 2002.

appetite or difficulty swallowing solids. For those fed via tube-based enteral nutrition, a change in the preparation to reflect the increased protein, vitamin, and mineral, as well as caloric, requirements is important.[10,12]

Treatment of incontinence with intermittent catheterization or changing schedule is helpful to reduce risk of skin breakdown. Placement of a urinary catheter may also be considered when a wound is present; however, this carries an increased risk of urinary tract infections.[4]

Prevention

Prevention of pressure ulcers in the primary care setting is best achieved by identifying patients at high risk. For bedbound patients, scheduled turning helps prevent pressure buildup in any one area. There is no clear guideline as to how often a patient needs to turn to avoid pressure buildup, but a schedule of every 2 hours is generally accepted.

For patients who are wheelchair bound, it is important to shift weight within the chair regularly, which can be achieved by shifting weight from side to side every few hours. Patients with adequate upper body strength, such as paraplegics, are taught to perform wheelchair push-ups in order to elevate the ischial area from the chair every few hours.[14]

Special population: athletes

Athletes with pressure ulcers are more common than might be expected. In one study, 87% of wheelchair-bound paralympic athletes reported either a current or previous pressure ulcer. Protecting these ulcers from further damage during competition is paramount. Choice of seating and cushion must allow the athlete to adequately propel the wheelchair for the sport but also must adequately relieve pressure from the injured area.[16]

Diabetic athletes with foot ulcers need to protect the injured area.[13,17] A period of partial weight bearing and limiting activity may be required. Finding appropriate shoes to prevent prolonged compression over high-pressure areas is important. There is some promise for custom insoles that are made after insole pressure testing, with the goal of minimizing foot pressures.[15] Athletes never want to take time off, which highlights the importance of helping these athletes find ways to cross-train while relieving pressure on their injured extremities.

Talon Noir

History
Also known as black heel or black dot heel, talon noir is hemorrhage into the skin from excess pressure to the sole of the foot or heel.[18,19] This condition is common in distance runners and jumpers, but is also seen in laborers who are on their feet for long periods of time. Repetitive microtrauma leads to papillary dermal hemorrhage, resulting in extravasation of blood under the stratum corneum (**Fig. 2**). Clinically this presents as asymptomatic, irregularly shaped, black or dark brown lesions. The history is key to making the diagnosis because this finding can mimic other diagnoses, including plantar wart and acral lentiginous melanoma.

Examination
A through history is usually sufficient for the correct diagnosis. If there is continued concern regarding the correct diagnosis, the lesion can be pared with a scalpel to reveal the hemorrhagic lesion that lies within the stratum corneum of the epidermis.[20] Pigmentation from melanoma cannot be removed by paring superficially within the epidermis.

Treatment
There is no specific treatment of this self-limited condition.

Prevention
Prevention of talon noir can be attempted by activity modification and by padding the heel to minimize trauma.

Corns and Calluses

History
Corns and calluses are hyperkeratotic lesions that develop as a result of repetitive pressure as a protective response. They are most commonly found on the feet but can occur in other areas subject to similar pressures.[18,21,22]

A corn is a well-circumscribed hyperkeratotic lesion that can cause pain and inflammation. Corns develop as a response to mechanical pressure over time. They result

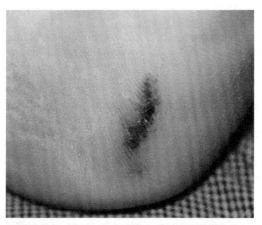

Fig. 2. Talon noir on the heel with extravasation of blood under the stratum corneum, as can be seen after repetitive heel strike in a runner. (*From* Schachner LA, Hansen RC. Physical injury and environmental hazards. In: Pediatric dermatology. 4th edition. Elsevier Mosby; 2011; with permission.)

from a thickening of the stratum corneum of the skin in the center of the hyperkeratotic lesion.

Calluses are broad areas of hyperkeratosis that develop in areas subjected to repeated mechanical pressure. They are not as well circumscribed as a corn. Along with the feet, calluses are often found on the hands of weight lifters, laborers, and participants in racquet sports. Calluses are desirable in many ways for athletes because they can allow continued participation without pain or injury. Therefore, treatment is rarely sought for these lesions.[23]

Examination

There are 2 types of corns: hard and soft. The more common hard corns are hyperkeratotic horns that form most commonly on the dorsum of the toes.[21]

Soft corns are less common. They result as the hyperkeratotic area becomes irritated and absorbs moisture, giving the corn a more chewed-up appearance. These corns are painful.

Evaluation of a callus reveals a broad area of hyperkeratosis that is less well defined. A callus is either a diffuse-shearing callus, which, as the name implies, is a diffuse area of hyperkeratosis, or a discrete nucleated callus, which is smaller and better circumscribed. The latter is often confused with a plantar wart, but debridement reveals a keratin plug, formed as a result of repeated mechanical stress. Calluses also retain their natural skin markings, distinguishing them from warts.

Treatment

Treatment of corns and calluses is symptomatic. The first step is modification of activity or equipment that may lead to the lesion. Footwear that evenly distributes pressure can be helpful. Shoes with a wide toe box minimize the pressure on the dorsum of the foot that leads to corns.[19,23]

Symptomatic treatment includes debridement or shaving of the callus or corn. Pumice can be used at home to pare down lesions that are not painful after soaking in warm water. For more painful lesions, sharp debridement in the office often provides relief. If a bony abnormality exists, surgical intervention may be required.[21]

Metatarsal pads are often effective for plantar callus formation. For calluses formed on the hands of laborers or weight lifters, padded gloves can provide relief and minimize stress. Racquet sport athletes often use tape over calluses to decrease pain or blister formation under the callus.

Occasionally surgical correction of a foot deformity that predisposes to callus or corn formation, such as hammer toe or claw toe deformities, may be necessary to prevent recurrence.

Prevention

Prevention of corns and calluses is best achieved by avoiding the pressures that result in their formation. Shoes with an adequate toe box prevent forces on the dorsal surface of the foot that often lead to corns.

FRICTION INJURIES
Intertrigo and Chafing

History

Intertrigo is inflammation that forms where there is chafing within skin folds because of moisture and friction. Chafing can also occur in areas of repetitive friction between body parts or equipment. Areas at risk for developing intertrigo are the diaper area in children and the groin and axilla in adults. Obese individuals are at risk in areas of excess skin folds.[24] Individuals who participate in endurance activities, such as runners, are susceptible to chafing in areas of increased friction, such as the inner thighs, or against equipment. The nipples of joggers and bikers are exposed to repetitive friction against clothing. This condition also occurs in surfers because of friction from board and wax.[18,19] On history, patients report mild erythema either in a skin fold or in an area of repetitive friction. Simple intertrigo is susceptible to bacterial or fungal superinfection. Patients with superinfection report increased erythema, spreading rash, and odor. Intertrigo presents similarly to other dermatologic conditions, such as contact dermatitis, atopic dermatitis, and inverse psoriasis, and these should be considered in the differential diagnosis.

Examination
Early cases of intertrigo present as erythematous patches or thin plaques in areas of friction. The erythema is often symmetrically distributed on either side of the skin fold.

Later in presentation there may be erosions, ulceration, oozing, and crusting. Signs of infection include malodor, maceration, and beefy redness, as seen in streptococcal cellulitis infections, as well as pustules and satellite lesions as seen in candida infection. Vital signs, especially temperature, are important in ruling out systemic manifestation of a local infection. Erythrasma infection is also common in intertriginous areas. This condition illuminates as coral red when examined with a Wood lamp. Pseudomonas infection can also present as intertrigo and illuminates green. Infection is more common in intertrigo than in chafing that is caused by repetitive activity, likely because of increased chronicity and moisture involved with intertrigo.

Treatment
Treatment of intertrigo includes reducing friction and moisture. Obese individuals should be encouraged to lose weight. In athletes and laborers who perform repetitive motions, use of nonconstricting and breathable clothing can minimize friction and sweating. Powder and barrier creams should be used to minimize moisture and friction respectively.

If there is significant inflammation present, a topical steroid cream or ointment can be considered. Candida or bacterial infections are not treated with topical steroids. Antifungal cream or powder or antibiotics (oral or topical) should be used depending on the findings on the physical examination, potassium hydroxide skin preparation, and/or available skin culture data.[25]

Prevention
Prevention of intertrigo and chafing involves minimizing friction in high-risk areas. Again, use of nonconstricting and breathable clothing can minimize friction and sweating in athletes and laborers. Powder or barrier creams are often helpful to prevent moisture. For endurance athletes, use of petroleum jelly over the inner thighs or nipples can prevent chafing in these high-risk areas.

Blisters

History
Blisters are caused by repetitive friction between the skin and an external surface.[19,26] These tender fluid-filled bullae occur secondary to repetitive friction resulting in a split within the layers of the epidermis. The uppermost layers of the skin remain intact, making the distal extremities the most common location given the thick skin of the palms and soles.[18] Most commonly, blisters result from friction between the foot or ankle and a piece of footwear. Blisters can also occur on the hands where they are in contact with a piece of equipment, such as a hammer in the hand of a construction worker.

A recent study showed that skin exposed to moisture showed a more rapid increase in temperature and thus was at increased risk of blister formation.[27]

Blisters commonly occur over a period of a few hours with repetitive friction. Patients with adequate sensation feel the blister forming. They often describe an area of heat or burning, frequently termed a hot spot. Modification of activity once a hot spot is noticed can stop progression to a blister. The hot spot is caused by an area of exfoliation of the stratum corneum. If unable to modify activity, then continued friction over the hot area causes separation of the skin at the level of the stratum spinosum, leading to the classic bullae formation. The space fills with fluid over time because of hydrostatic pressure.

Examination

The classic presentation of a blister is a bulla filled with clear fluid. Occasionally, a blister fills with blood and is dark brownish in color. An infected blister may be filled with pus. Often, by the time the patient is seen in the office, the blister has ruptured. Then, the roof is collapsed against the underlying skin. The area is often tender to palpation.

The area should be inspected for signs of infection. It is also important to identify the underlying cause of the blister. For blisters on the feet, it may be helpful to examine footwear.

Treatment

Treatment of a blister includes local skin care and modification of activity or stresses.

Small, nontense blisters do not require drainage. The epidermal roof is helpful in preventing infection. Large or tense blisters can be drained to reduce pressure and pain as well as to decrease expansion of the blister. A sterile needle or scalpel can be used to place a small puncture hole into the epidermal roof allowing the fluid to drain outward. As much of the roof as possible should be maintained and allowed to collapse onto the underlying skin, to provide a barrier against infection (**Fig. 3**). Once drained the area can be covered with a transparent gel or hydrocolloid type of dressing to protect the area and decrease further friction. Many blister dressings are sold over the counter.

The best approach for blister healing is activity modification until healing has occurred.

Prevention

Reducing friction by changing equipment or applying padding, such as moleskin, helps in healing and preventing blisters. Powders and moisture-wicking clothing

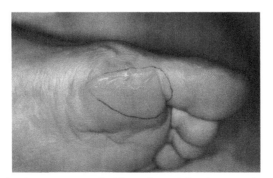

Fig. 3. Blister that has been punctured with roof remaining intact and overlying the round. (*From* Mailler-Savage EA, Adams BB. Skin manifestations of running. J Am Acad Dermatol 2006;55(2):290–301; with permission.)

(acrylic and/or polyester) can reduce risk by decreasing moisture. Wet socks should be changed often. Petroleum jelly or similar substances may reduce friction in high-risk areas.

For patients with decreased sensation, it is important to examine new equipment and footwear frequently because these individuals cannot sense a hot spot and progress rapidly to blister formation, which can lead to further skin breakdown and ulceration.[13,17]

Abrasions

History

Acute abrasions are common and, in most patients, do not require medical attention. Abrasions occur when a sudden shearing or friction force causes abrupt separation of the superficial keratinized area of skin from the underlying skin. This separation may expose the lower epidermis, or, in more significant abrasions, the papillary dermis. This condition usually leads to an area of small capillary destruction leading to pinpoint bleeding that appears as an area of reddened skin. These abrasions are commonly referred to as raspberries because of their similarity in appearance. Abrasions are often noticed as a secondary issue when a patient presents after a fall or accident (eg, road rash in cycling). In many sports, abrasions are caused by repetitive friction. Jogger's nipples are a classic example presenting in long-distance runners. The nipples become painful, red, and eroded from repetitive rubbing of coarse fabric against the breasts. Turf burns are abrasions secondary to friction with artificial turf or grass, and swimmer's shoulder is caused by repeated friction with a male swimmer's unshaven beard.[23]

Examination

The size and depth should be noted on examination of the abrasion. The presence of pus, weeping, or honey-colored crusting indicates infection. Examination of the abrasion should also include a search for foreign matter, such as debris from the road or field where the injury occurred.[18]

Treatment

Treatment of abrasions is supportive. A dirty wound should be aggressively irrigated with saline or sterile water. Cleaning with cytotoxic agents such as hydrogen peroxide is not encouraged. Application of white petroleum jelly or an antibacterial cream is adequate for protection after cleansing of small abrasions. Deeper or larger abrasions may require covering with a transparent gel or hydrocolloid, to maintain moisture and provide a barrier of protection (see **Table 4**). For athletes and laborers, the area needs to be protected against friction and a padded dressing should be applied to cover the wound. For minor abrasions, healing is usually complete within 7 to 14 days and long-term scarring is rare.[18]

Prevention

Prevention of abrasions is difficult because these often occur suddenly as a result of a fall or accident. High-risk areas in athletes or laborers should be padded. Children can be encouraged to wear elbow and knee pads while riding bikes and skateboards.

Acne Mechanica

History

Formation of pustules or papules in areas of friction from equipment or padding is referred to as acne mechanica. This inflammatory condition occurs from the moisture and repetitive friction under such equipment. The shoulders or chests of football players wearing shoulder pads are a common location (**Fig. 4**). It is also seen under

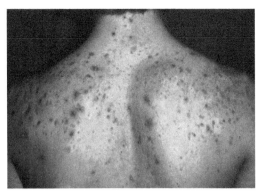

Fig. 4. Acne mechanica after repetitive friction caused by shoulder pads in the setting of preexisting acne vulgaris. (*From* Marchetti MA, Wilson B. Dermatologic conditions. In: Miller MD, Thompson SR, eds. DeLee & Drez's orthopaedic sports medicine. Philadelphia: Elsevier Saunders; 2015. p. 285–97; with permission.)

chin straps and sports bras. Truck drivers may be at risk on their backs because of vibration of the truck.

Examination

Patients present with a complaint of acne in an area of friction. Inspection reveals inflammatory pustules or papules. More chronic cases may have scarring or cystic changes. Bacterial superinfection in the form of impetigo can occur, so inspection should be performed for weeping or crusting lesions.

Treatment

Ultimate treatment of acne mechanica is removal of the friction-causing agent.[28] After removal of the cause for a few days the lesions usually start to subside. If removal of the agent is not possible then modifications to reduce moisture and friction should be encouraged. Patients who perspire heavily should be encouraged to change their undergarments frequently. Moisture-wicking clothing (including cotton) and powders can be helpful to reduce moisture. Alteration of straps or padding to reduce friction should also be tried. The area should be washed immediately after each workout. Benzoyl peroxide may be helpful to prevent follicular occlusion, and antibiotics, such as oral doxycycline, may be helpful if acne is widespread.

Prevention

Prevention of acne mechanica can be achieved by the use of moisture-wicking clothing, and powders to prevent moisture. Petroleum jelly can prevent friction. For athletes or individuals who have a history of acne mechanica, education on preventing moisture and friction, including changing of clothing on a scheduled basis, may be helpful.

SUMMARY

Pressure and friction injuries to the skin are commonly encountered by primary care providers. Pressure ulcers are common in debilitated patients and treatment is best with a multidisciplinary approach. Most other pressure and friction injuries should be treated with modification of activity and supportive care.

Because the skin is the body's natural barrier, improper care of these injuries may lead to infection.

REFERENCES

1. Blackwell DL, Lucas JW, Clarke TC. Summary health statistics for U.S. adults: National Health Interview Survey, 2012. National Center for Health Statistics. Vital Health Stat 2014;10(260):1–161.
2. Lowell BA, Froelich CW, Federman DG, et al. Dermatology in primary care: prevalence and patient disposition. J Am Acad Dermatol 2001;45(2):250–5.
3. Leijon S, Bergh I, Terstappen K. Pressure ulcer prevalence, use of preventive measures, and mortality risk in an acute care population: a quality improvement project. J Wound Ostomy Continence Nurs 2013;40(5):469–74.
4. National Pressure Ulcer Advisory Panel and European Pressure Ulcer Advisory Panel. Prevention and treatment of pressure ulcer: clinical practice guideline. Washington, DC: National Pressure Ulcer Advisory Panel; 2009.
5. Bluestein D, Javaheri A. Pressure ulcers: prevention, evaluation, and management. Am Fam Physician 2008;78(10):1186–94.
6. Stotts NA, Rodeheaver G, Thomas DR, et al. An instrument to measure healing in pressure ulcers: development and validation of the Pressure Ulcer Scale for Healing (PUSH). J Gerontol A Biol Sci Med Sci 2001;56(12):M795–9.
7. Dorner B, Posthauer ME, Thomas D, National Pressure Ulcer Advisory Panel. The role of nutrition in pressure ulcer prevention and treatment: National Pressure Ulcer Advisory Panel white paper. Adv Skin Wound Care 2009;22(5):212–21.
8. Yatabe MS, Taguchi F, Ishida I, et al. Mini nutritional assessment as a useful method of predicting the development of pressure ulcers in elderly inpatients. J Am Geriatr Soc 2013;61(10):1698–704.
9. Hess CT. Wound care. 4th edition. Springhouse (PA): Springhouse; 2002.
10. Langer G, Fink A. Nutritional interventions for preventing and treating pressure ulcers. Cochrane Database Syst Rev 2014;(6):CD003216.
11. VanGilder C, MacFarlane G, Meyer S, et al. Body mass index, weight, and pressure ulcer prevalence: an analysis of the 2006–2007 international pressure ulcer prevalence surveys. J Nurs Care Qual 2009;24(2):127–35.
12. Cereda E, Klersy C, Serioli M, et al. A nutritional formula enriched with arginine, zinc, and antioxidants for the healing of pressure ulcers: a randomized trial. Ann Intern Med 2015;162(3):167–74.
13. Waaijman R, de Haart M, Arts ML, et al. Risk factors for plantar foot ulcer recurrence in neuropathic diabetic patients. Diabetes Care 2014;37(6):1697–705.
14. Makhsous M, Rowles DM, Rymer WZ, et al. Periodically relieving ischial sitting load to decrease the risk of pressure ulcers. Arch Phys Med Rehabil 2007; 88(7):862–70.
15. Ulbrecht JS, Hurley T, Mauger DT, et al. Prevention of recurrent foot ulcers with plantar pressure-based in-shoe orthoses: the CareFUL prevention multicenter randomized controlled trial. Diabetes Care 2014;37(7):1982–9.
16. Miller SL. Medical aspects of paralympic sport. Sportex Med 2009;42:13–9.
17. Lavery LA, Baranoski S, Ayello EA. Options for off-loading the diabetic foot. Adv Skin Wound Care 2004;17:181–6.
18. Adams BB. Dermatologic disorders of the athlete. Sports Med 2002;32(5):309–21.
19. Basler RS, Hunzeker CM, Garcia MA. Athletic skin injuries: combating pressure and friction. Phys Sportsmed 2004;32(5):33–40.
20. Googe AB, Schulmeier JS, Jackson AR, et al. Talon noir: paring can eliminate the need for a biopsy. Postgrad Med J 2014;90:730–1.
21. Freeman DP. Corns and calluses resulting from mechanical hyperkeratosis. Am Fam Physician 2002;65(11):2277–80.

22. Spink MJ, Menz HB, Lord SR. Distribution of plantar hyperkeratotic lesions in older people. J Foot Ankle Res 2009;2:8.

23. Cordoro KM, Ganz JE. Training room management of medical conditions: sports dermatology. Clin Sports Med 2005;24:565–98.

24. Yosipovitch G, DeVore A, Dawn A. Obesity and the skin: skin physiology and skin manifestations of obesity. J Am Acad Dermatol 2007;56(6):901–16.

25. Kalra MG, Higgins KE, Kinney BS. Intertrigo and secondary skin infections. Am Fam Physician 2014;89(7):569–73.

26. De Luca JF, Adams BB, Yosipovitch G. Skin manifestations of athletes competing in the Summer Olympics: what a sports medicine physician should know. Sports Med 2012;42(5):399–413.

27. Kirkham S, Lam S, Nester C, et al. The effect of hydration on the risk of friction blister formation on the heel of the foot. Skin Res Technol 2014;20(2):246–53.

28. Kang YC, Choi EH, Hwang SM, et al. Acne mechanica due to an orthopedic crutch. Cutis 1999;64(2):97–8.

Skin Cancer

Miguel A. Linares, MD[a], Alan Zakaria, DO, MS[b],
Parminder Nizran, MD, CCFP[c],*

KEYWORDS

- Basal cell carcinoma • Squamous cell carcinoma • Melanoma • Dermoscopy
- Excision margin • Melanonychia • Histopathologic

KEY POINTS

- Cancer of the skin is the most common type of cancer in humans. Melanoma accounts for only 2% of all skin cancers but causes most skin cancer deaths.
- Melanoma is more than 20 times more common in white people than in African Americans. Individuals with fair skin and chronic sun exposure are at the highest risk for melanoma but other factors also contribute to the overall risk.
- Definitive diagnosis of skin malignancy is usually made with skin biopsy and histopathologic examination; history and physical examination are key components to diagnosing skin malignancies. Skin biopsy types include excisional biopsy, punch biopsy, and shave biopsy.
- Dermoscopy seems to increase sensitivity in detecting skin cancers and a working knowledge of this modality can be helpful in the primary care setting.
- Prevention measures include the appropriate use of sunscreen, minimizing sun exposure, wearing hats and long clothing while exposed to the sun, and avoiding tanning beds.

INTRODUCTION

Skin cancer is the most common form of cancer in the United States. Most skin cancers are nonmelanomatous. Malignant nonmelanoma skin cancers originate from keratinized epithelial cells. These cancers include basal cell carcinoma (BCC) and squamous cell carcinoma (SCC). Melanoma only accounts for about 2% of malignant skin cancer but causes most deaths. More than 2 million cases of skin cancer were diagnosed in the United States in 2010. BCC is the most common form and is usually slow growing and locally invasive. SCC is the second most common form of nonmelanomatous skin cancer, accounting for approximately 20% to 30% of cases.[1–3]

Disclosure: The authors have nothing to disclose.
[a] Primary Care Sports Medicine Fellow, Henry Ford Hospital, 2799 W Grand Boulevard, Detroit, MI 48208, USA; [b] Nahed A. Zakaria MD, P.C., 1080 Kirts Boulevard, Ste #400, Troy, MI 48084, USA; [c] Albion Family Clinic & Walkin, Unit 309-1620, Albion Road, Etobicoke, ON M9V4B4, Canada
* Corresponding author.
E-mail address: parmindermd@hotmail.com

Prim Care Clin Office Pract 42 (2015) 645–659
http://dx.doi.org/10.1016/j.pop.2015.07.006
0095-4543/15/$ – see front matter © 2015 Elsevier Inc. All rights reserved.

primarycare.theclinics.com

The most important risk factor is chronic ultraviolet exposure. Diagnosis is usually suspected in older, fair-skinned individuals with scaly, indurated lesions on sun-exposed areas, primarily on the head and neck. Accuracy of clinical diagnosis can be enhanced using magnification, adequate lighting, and a dermatoscope. Biopsy with histopathologic confirmation is required for definitive diagnosis. Full-thickness biopsy is required for evaluation of melanoma because management and prognosis depend on the depth of the lesion. Overall cases of all forms of skin cancers have been increasing across the world.

Some studies have shown an increase in melanoma incidence among young individuals, with some epidemiologic studies showing as much as a 50% incidence in individuals aged 35 to 65 years. Working knowledge of these common malignancies is important in primary care settings. If there is a suspicion of a skin cancer lesion, a biopsy should be performed or a referral to a dermatologist should be initiated.

SKIN BIOPSY
Indication to Biopsy

- Suspected neoplastic lesions
- Bullous disorders
- If diagnosis is unclear and/or for therapeutic purposes

Contraindications to Biopsy

Contraindications to biopsy include infected site (if diagnosis of infection is not what is being considered), bleeding disorders, and patients on blood thinners.

Patients should not be taken off therapeutic or prophylactic blood thinners for a skin biopsy. These patients may benefit from being referred to a dermatologist if it is thought that hemostasis will be a problem. Lesions on the face, eyelids, and lips may need to be referred to a dermatologist or plastic surgeon because they are in readily visible locations.

Patients should be asked about allergies to topical antibiotics, antiseptics, local anesthetics, and tape, as well as bleeding disorders and any use of blood-thinning medications.

Site Selection

- Thickest, most pigmented area
- Area with most inflammatory changes
- For blistering lesions, a newly formed vesicle should be chosen
- Bullae should be biopsied at their edge

Types of Skin Biopsy

- Punch
- Shave
- Excision

Punch Biopsy

- Not a sterile procedure
- The site should be prepared with isopropyl alcohol, povidone-iodine, or chlorhexidine
- The site should be anesthetized with 1% to 2% lidocaine
- Epinephrine may be added to lidocaine if the site is not at the digits, ears, or nose
- A disposable round knife punch may be used
- May be used to excise small lesions

- Size ranges from 2 mm to 10 mm
- Biopsy is taken to the depth of the subcutaneous tissue
- Skin may heal by secondary intention
- Either 1 or 2 sutures may be used for better cosmetic results in larger punch biopsies
- Single-layer simple interrupted sutures are adequate
- Patients should be instructed to keep the area clean and to apply ointment such as bacitracin twice daily
- Biopsies not sutured should be covered with clean gauze and changed twice daily

Shave Biopsy

- Not a sterile procedure
- The site should be prepared with isopropyl alcohol, povidone-iodine, or chlorhexidine
- The site may be anesthetized with 1% to 2% lidocaine
- Wheal of anesthesia may be used to raise the lesion to aid the ease of the biopsy
- May add epinephrine to lidocaine if the site is not at the digits, ears, or nose
- Performed with 15-blade scalpel or double-edged razor
- Ideal for raised lesions and lesions confined to the epidermis
- This technique should not be used for a pigmented lesion or a lesion suspicious for melanoma
- Sutures are not necessary
- May leave a depressed scar once healed
- Patients should be instructed to keep area clean and apply ointments such as bacitracin twice daily
- The biopsy site should be covered with gauze and changed twice daily after cleaning

Excisional Biopsy

- Sterile procedure
- The site should be prepared with isopropyl alcohol, povidone-iodine, or chlorhexidine
- The site may be anesthetized site with 1% to 2% lidocaine
- Epinephrine may be added to lidocaine if the site is not at the digits, ears, or nose
- Performed with a scalpel
- Biopsy is taken to the depth of the subcutaneous tissue
- Ideal for lesions that are large, known to be malignant, or are typical of a malignancy
- Sutures are necessary
- Patients should be instructed to keep the area clean and apply ointments such as bacitracin twice daily

BASAL CELL CARCINOMA

BCC is a skin cancer that originates from the basal layer of the epidermis and its appendages. It is caused by cell mutations induced by ultraviolet radiation and thus arises most commonly on sun-exposed areas, such as the nose, ears, face, and backs of hands; however, it may occur anywhere on the body. It is a slow-growing cancer that rarely metastasizes.

Epidemiology

It is estimated by the American Cancer Society that approximately 3.5 million nonmelanoma skin cancers were treated in the United States in 2006. It is thought that 80% or greater of these skin cancers were BCC. This cancer is more common among white people and the incidence in men is 30% higher than in women. The lifetime risk of developing BCC is 30%. The incidence of BCC increases with age and proximity to the equator. Approximately 40% of individuals diagnosed with BCC develop another lesion within 5 years.[4–6]

Risk Factors

Risk factors for BCC are identical to those of other skin cancers (sun exposure, fair complexion, light eyes) but also include:

- Ionizing radiation
- Chronic arsenic exposure
- Basal cell nevus syndrome (Gorlin syndrome), which is an autosomal dominant mutation of the human patched gene

Clinical Presentation

BCC can be divided into 3 main subtypes: superficial, nodular, and morpheaform. The nodular variant makes up approximately 60% of cases, superficial BCC accounts for another 30%, and morpheaform BCC occurs 5% to 10%. Each group has its own distinct physical characteristics and histologic findings.[1,6–8]

Nodular Basal Cell Carcinoma

Nodular BCC most commonly presents on the face as a pearly, skin-colored, or pink papule. The papule typically has a translucent pearly appearance, telangiectasias, and may have ulceration (**Fig. 1**).

Superficial Basal Cell Carcinoma

Superficial BCC typically appears on the trunk, presenting as an erythematous, scaly papule or plaque. The border of the lesion may be lined with translucent papules and the center of the lesion may appear atrophic (**Fig. 2**).

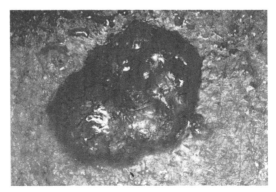

Fig. 1. Nodular BCC.

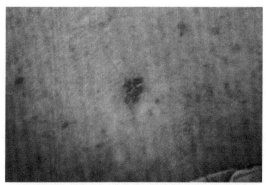

Fig. 2. Superficial BCC. (*From* National Cancer Institute/Kelly Nelson. Basal cell carcinoma, superficial. Available at: https://visualsonline.cancer.gov/details.cfm?imageid=9236.)

Morpheaform Basal Cell Carcinoma

Morpheaform BCC presents as an erythematous or skin-colored papule or plaque. The lesion may appear scarlike with induration, atrophy, and irregular borders (**Fig. 3**).

Treatment

BCC is easily treated in the outpatient setting. Electrodessication and curettage or local excision is curative. Mohs micrographic surgery may be used in cosmetically

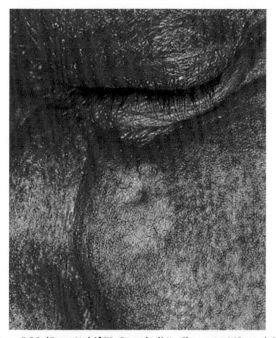

Fig. 3. Morpheaform BCC. (*From* Habif TP, Campbell JL, Chapman MS, et al. Premalignant and malignant non-melanoma skin tumors. In: Gabbery R, editor. Skin disease. 3rd edition. Philadelphia: Saunders; 2011. p. 470; with permission.)

sensitive areas such as eyelids, ears, nose, and lips, or for larger or recurrent lesions. Topical imiquimod 5% cream can also be used to treat superficial BCC.[9]

SQUAMOUS CELL CARCINOMA

Cutaneous SCC arises from malignant, uncontrolled proliferation of epidermal keratinocytes. Like BCC, SCC is also caused largely by ultraviolet radiation.

Epidemiology

Cutaneous SCC is the second most common skin cancer. The exact percentage of cutaneous SCC cases in the United States is not known because they are usually not reported to cancer registries. The incidence of SCC in the United States is estimated to be around 20% of nonmelanoma skin cancer cases.[1,7]

Bowen Disease

Bowen disease is the intraepithelial form of SCC, also known as SCC in situ. Bowen is associated with human papillomavirus in addition to typical skin cancer risk factors. It is confined to the epidermis and does not infiltrate the dermis. It presents as a rough, scaly, erythematous plaque with irregular borders. Most cases present on the lower legs and sun-exposed skin, and are found in women. However, this lesion can appear in any location. Because Bowen disease is confined to the epidermis, unlike invasive SCC, effective treatment can be seen with cryotherapy, cauterization, and topical 5-fluorouracil.

Erythroplasia of Queyrat

Erythroplasia of Queyrat is a form of SCC in situ that presents on the glans or prepuce of the penis in men and the vulvae in women. Like Bowen disease, the atypical malignant squamous cells are confined to the thickness of the epidermis. This condition is associated with the human papillomavirus. For this reason, erythroplasia of Queyrat is also called Bowen disease of the glans penis. The lesion presents as an erythematous scaly or crusting plaque that may have bleeding and/or ulceration. Cases are almost exclusively seen in middle-aged uncircumcised men. Effective treatment is readily achieved with the same modalities as in Bowen disease.

Risk Factors

Risk factors for SCC are identical to those of BCC but also include the following:

- Chronic inflammation caused by a laceration, scar, burn, ulcer, or other skin damage
- Epidermolysis bullosa syndromes (a group of skin diseases that make individuals prone to forming bullae on the skin without a traumatic event to the skin)

Clinical Presentation

Similar to other skin cancers, SCC most commonly presents on sun-exposed areas, but can develop anywhere on the body. SCC commonly presents as rough, erythematous papules, plaques, and nodules with well-demarcated borders and crusting. The lesions may show ulceration, pigmentation, erythema, scaling, or hyperkeratosis (**Fig. 4**).

Diagnosis

A diagnosis is made via biopsy of the lesion and histopathologic examination. Shave, punch, or excisional biopsies are all acceptable methods for suspected SCC diagnosis.

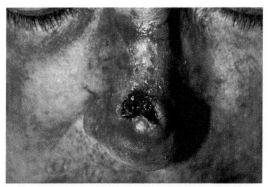

Fig. 4. SCC. (*From* Squamous cell carcinoma. National Cancer Institute. Available at: https://visualsonline.cancer.gov/details.cfm?imageid=2165.)

Treatment

Treatment of SCC is similar to that of BCC and can be handled in an outpatient setting. Because of the increased risk for metastasis, surgical excision or Mohs surgery is preferred to electrodessication and curettage. Surgical excision should be performed with a goal of a margin of 4 mm to 6 mm. Radiation therapy is an option for larger cancers or in patients who are not candidates for surgical intervention.

Risk Factors for Recurrence of Cutaneous Squamous Cell Carcinoma

- Location
- Size
- Poorly defined borders
- Recurrent tumors
- Immunosuppressed patient
- Site of previous radiation therapy or chronic inflammation
- Rapidly growing tumor
- Neurologic symptoms
- Moderately or poorly differentiated tumor
- Adenoid, adenosquamous, or desmoplastic subtypes
- Depth greater than or equal to 2 mm or Clark level IV–V[9]
- Perineural or vascular involvement

MELANOMA

Melanoma is an aggressive malignant neoplasm derived from melanocytes. Melanocytes are found in the basal layer of the epidermis. When they are exposed to ultraviolet light there is an accumulation of genetic mutations that activate oncogenes, inactivate tumor suppressor genes, and impair DNA repair. This process may lead to uncontrolled proliferation of melanocytes and ultimately melanoma.

For patients with cutaneous melanoma, the prognosis is related to the location and depth of the primary tumor, and the presence or absence of localized and distant metastatic disease.

There are 4 major subtypes of invasive cutaneous melanoma that are grouped for their distinct histologic patterns: superficial, nodular, lentigo maligna, and acral lentiginous.

Epidemiology

Estimates for 2014 are that 76,100 invasive melanomas will be diagnosed in the United States and that melanoma could claim 9710 lives. Melanoma is the fifth most common cancer in men and the seventh in women in the United States.

The incidence rates for invasive melanoma among white individuals in the United States in the years 2006 to 2010 were 27.4 per 100,000 men and 16.7 per 100,000 women per year (**Fig. 5**). From 1992 to 2006, the incidence increased by more than 3% per year among non-Hispanic white people. The increase was observed in both sexes and in all age groups and was highest in individuals aged 65 years and older.[7]

Superficial Melanoma

Superficial melanoma is the most common subtype and makes up 75% of malignant melanomas. Histologic findings in this subgroup are a radial growth before growing vertically into deeper tissue layers. During this radial growth phase the melanoma spreads by single-cell dispersal. Once nests of neoplastic melanocytes reach past the papillary dermis and the dermal layer the lesion is considered to be in its vertical growth phase. Superficial melanoma occurs more frequently on the backs in men and the lower extremities in women. The lesion may present with variable colors (black, blue, brown, white, gray, red), irregular borders, and an asymmetric flare at the lesion's border that represents the advancing proliferation of melanocytes (**Fig. 6**).[4,10,11]

Nodular Melanoma

Nodular melanoma is an aggressive, vertically growing melanoma that comprises 15% to 30% of melanomas. It does not have a radial growth phase, thus growing in depth more quickly than in width. For this reason, it may take longer for a person to be suspicious of the lesion. Nodular melanoma commonly present as darkly pigmented pedunculated or polypoid nodules (**Fig. 7**).

Lentigo Maligna Melanoma

Lentigo maligna melanoma is the second most common subtype of melanoma. It most commonly presents on sun-exposed areas as a small, flat, tan, irregular-bordered, asymmetric macule that, over time, enlarges and begins to vary in color (**Fig. 8**).

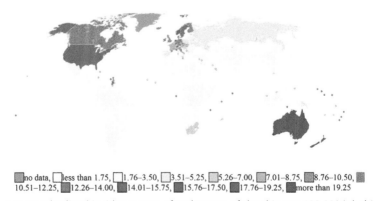

no data, less than 1.75, 1.76–3.50, 3.51–5.25, 5.26–7.00, 7.01–8.75, 8.76–10.50, 10.51–12.25, 12.26–14.00, 14.01–15.75, 15.76–17.50, 17.76–19.25, more than 19.25

Fig. 5. Age-standardized incidence rate of melanoma of the skin per 100,000 inhabitants in 2008.

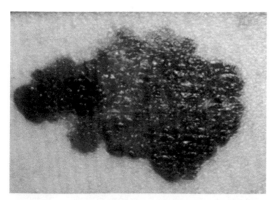

Fig. 6. Superficial melanoma. (*From* National Cancer Institute (AV number: AV-8500-3850; date created: 1985; date entered: 1/1/2001). Available at: http://visualsonline.cancer.gov/details.cfm?imageid=2184.)

Acral Lentiginous

Acral lentiginous melanoma most commonly appears in palmar, plantar, and subungual locations (**Fig. 9**). This melanoma is the least common subtype and accounts for fewer than 5% of cases. However, compared with white people, the rates in Asians, Chinese, Japanese, African, and Middle Eastern people is significantly higher.[12,13]

Subungual melanoma most commonly presents as longitudinal melanonychia, which is a black or brown pigmentation of the normal nail plate (**Fig. 10**). The added involvement of the proximal nail fold, known as Hutchinson sign, is also an indicator of a malignant cause. Transverse melanonychia without Hutchinson sign suggests a benign cause. Melanonychia may be a normal finding in dark-skinned individuals as a result of trauma, or a postinflammatory event.

Melanonychia Differential

- Chronic paronychia
- Onychomycosis
- Subungual hematoma
- Pyogenic granuloma
- Glomus tumor
- Subungual verruca
- Mucous cyst

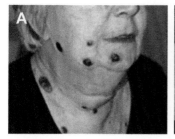
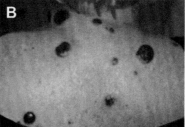

Fig. 7. Nodular melanoma. (*From* Rathi VK, Williams RB, Yamrozik J, et al. Cardiovascular magnetic resonance of the charcoal heart. J Cardiovasc Magn Reson 2008;10:37.)

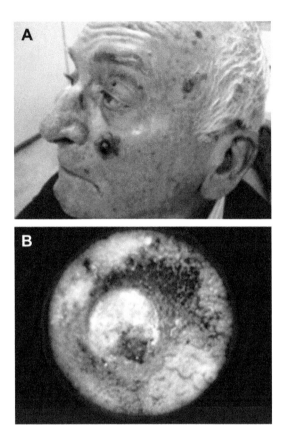

Fig. 8. (*A*) Histologically confirmed lentigo maligna melanoma on left cheek of an elderly male patient, arising from a lentigo maligna after many years. (*B*) Dermoscopic view of lentigo maligna melanoma. (*From* Tsatsou F, Trakatelli M, Patsatsi A, et al. Extrinsic aging: UV-mediated skin carcinogenesis. Dermatoendocrinol 2012;4(3):295.)

- Subungual fibroma
- Keratoacanthoma

Risk Factors

Risk factors for melanoma include:

- The presence of a high number of common nevi
- One or more atypical nevi
- Light skin
- Excessive sun exposure
- History of sunburns
- Tanning bed exposure
- Older age
- Family history in first-degree relatives

Clinical Presentation

Nevi that have the following characteristics (**Fig. 11**):

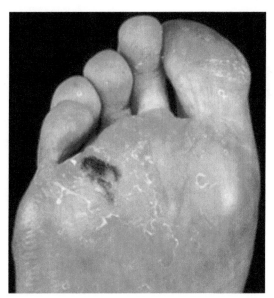

Fig. 9. Acral lentiginous melanoma on the plantar surface. (*From* Bristow IR, Acland K. Acral lentiginous melanoma of the foot and ankle: a case series and review of the literature. J Foot Ankle Res 2008;1(1):11.)

- Asymmetry
- Irregular borders
- Variegated color
- Diameter greater than 6 mm
- Recent change including size color and shape
- Inflammation

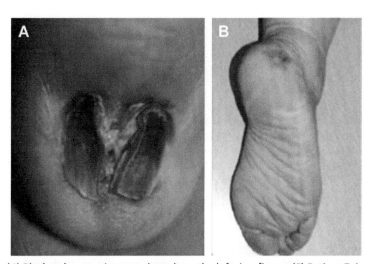

Fig. 10. (*A*) Black to brown pigmented patch on the left ring finger. (*B*) Patient 7: irregularly pigmented patch on the right heel. (*From* Park HS, Cho KH. Acral lentiginous melanoma in situ: a diagnostic and management challenge. Cancers (Basel). 2010;2(2):643.)

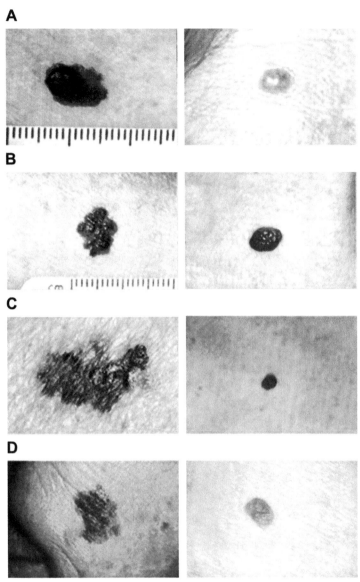

Fig. 11. ABCD rule. Melanomas showing (*A*) asymmetry; (*B*) a border that is uneven, ragged, or notched; (*C*) coloring of different shades of brown, black, or tan; and (*D*) diameter that had changed in size. The normal moles on the right side do not have abnormal characteristics (no asymmetry, even border, even color, no change in diameter).

- Bleeding or crusting
- Sensory change

When evaluating patients with multiple nevi it may be helpful to use the so-called ugly-duckling sign. This sign is based on the observation that nevi, although numerous, all tend to have a similar morphology. However, a lesion with a different morphology from surrounding lesions should be considered suspicious.

Using a dermatoscope to further evaluate the characteristics of a lesion in the clinical setting may be of some use (**Fig. 12**). However, the help it may provide in detecting melanoma is limited by the operator's training in dermoscopy. A meta-analysis of dermoscopy examinations compared with naked-eye examination in the diagnosis of melanoma concluded that, for clinicians with at least some training in dermoscopy, the addition of dermoscopy to the unaided clinical examination increases the sensitivity in detecting melanoma (90% vs 71%), but has similar specificity (80% vs 90%).

Diagnosis

Histopathology is the gold standard of diagnosis. A biopsy should be performed of any lesion that is suspected to be melanoma. If it is unclear whether a lesion is benign or if indication for biopsy is unclear the patient should be referred to a dermatologist. An excisional biopsy that includes the entire lesion with 1-mm to 3-mm margins of normal skin and part of the subcutaneous fat should be performed whenever possible. A shave biopsy should not be used if melanoma is suspected because the depth of the lesion is vital for staging purposes. An excisional biopsy has the added benefit of being diagnostic as well as therapeutic.

Treatment

Once a diagnosis has been made by biopsy of the lesion, pathologic staging must be completed to determine prognosis and treatment. Staging is as follows:

- Stage 0 (in situ): melanoma confined to the epidermis; recommended excision margin, 0.5 to 1 cm
- Stage I: less than or equal to 1 mm thick; 10-year survival, 92%; recommended excision margin, 1 cm
- Stage II: 1.01 to 4.00 mm thick; 10-year survival, 80%; recommended excision margin, 2 cm
- Stage III: melanoma has spread to nearby lymph node; 10-year survival, 63%
- Stage IV: melanoma has spread to an internal organ, lymph node far from the original melanoma, or is found on the skin far from the original melanoma; 10-year survival, 50%[14]

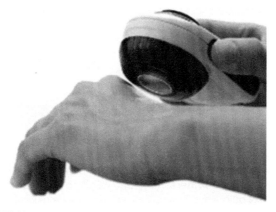

Fig. 12. Dermatoscope.

A sentinel lymph node biopsy should be considered for patients with primary melanoma larger than 1 mm or a primary melanoma smaller than 1 mm with negative prognostic features.

Monitoring

At present there are no randomized trials to evaluate screening effectiveness. A 2009 update from the United States Preventive Services Task Force found insufficient evidence to recommend for or against either routine screening of the general population for skin cancer by primary care providers or counseling patients to perform periodic skin self-examinations.

The American Academy of Dermatology recommends that those at highest risk, having a strong family history of melanoma and multiple atypical moles, should perform frequent self-examination and seek professional evaluation of the skin at least once per year.

Skin Cancer Prevention

Prevention is focused on proper protection from the sun whenever possible. Proper protection includes:

- Sun avoidance
- Full-length clothing that covers exposed skin
- Hats and sunglasses
- Use of broad-spectrum (ultraviolet A/ultraviolet B) sunscreen and sunblock with frequent reapplications
- Avoiding tanning bed exposure

It is vital that discussion of skin cancer prevention is incorporated into the counseling of patients at all well-child and adult wellness visits.

REFERENCES

1. American Cancer Society Cancer facts and figures 2010. Available at: http://www.cancer.org/acs/groups/content/@epidemiologysurveilance/documents/document/acspc-026238.pdf. Accessed October 4, 2010.
2. Miller DL, Weinstock MA. Nonmelanoma skin cancer in the United States: incidence. J Am Acad Dermatol 1994;30(5 Pt 1):774.
3. American Cancer Society. Cancer facts and figures 2003. Available at: whyquit.com/studies/2003_acs_cancer_facts.pdf. Accessed April 01, 2004.
4. American Academy of Dermatology and AAD Association; melanoma fact sheet. Available at: http://www.aad.org/public/exams/screenings/documents/AAD_Melanoma_Fact_Sheet.pdf. Accessed January 21, 2011.
5. Robinson JK. Risk of developing another basal cell carcinoma. A 5-year prospective study. Cancer 1987;60:118.
6. Karagas MR, Stukel TA, Greenberg ER, et al. Risk of subsequent basal cell carcinoma and squamous cell carcinoma of the skin among patients with prior skin cancer. Skin Cancer Prevention Study Group. JAMA 1992;267:3305.
7. Siegel R, Ma J, Zou Z, et al. Cancer statistics, 2014. CA Cancer J Clin 2014;64(1):9.
8. US Preventive Services Task Force. Screening for skin cancer: U.S. Preventive Services Task Force recommendation statement. Ann Intern Med 2009;150(3):188.
9. Bichakjian CK, Alam M, Andersen J, et al. NCCN clinical practice guidelines in oncology (NCCN guidelines): basal cell and squamous cell skin cancers, version I.2013. National Comprehensive Cancer Network; 2013.

10. Abbasi NR, Shaw HM, Rigel DS, et al. Early diagnosis of cutaneous melanoma: revisiting the ABCD criteria. JAMA 2004;292(22):2771.

11. Vestergaard ME, Macaskill P, Holt PE, et al. Dermoscopy compared with naked eye examination for the diagnosis of primary melanoma: a meta-analysis of studies performed in a clinical setting. Br J Dermatol 2008; 159(3):669.

12. Bristow IR, Acland K. Acral lentiginous melanoma of the foot and ankle: a case series and review of the literature. J Foot Ankle Res 2008;1(1):11.

13. Park HS, Cho KH. Acral lentiginous melanoma in situ: a diagnostic and management challenge. Cancers (Basel) 2010;2(2):642–52.

14. Edge S, Byrd DR, Compton CC, et al, editors. AJCC cancer staging manual. 7th edition. New York: Springer-Verlag; 2010. p. 299–340.

Parasitic Skin Infections for Primary Care Physicians

Irfan Dadabhoy, MD[a,1], Jessica F. Butts, MD[b,c],*

KEYWORDS

- Epidermal parasitic skin infections • Scabies • Pediculosis • Lice

KEY POINTS

- Scabies:
  - Presentation: diffuse pruritus and skin rash, often featuring burrows.
  - First-line treatment is topical permethrin or oral ivermectin.
- Pediculosis capitis:
  - Presentation: pruritus of scalp, neck, and outer ear.
  - Adult lice or nits may be found in scalp/hair.
  - Treatments of choice are topical pediculicides.
- Pediculosis pubis:
  - Presentation: pruritus in the pubic area.
  - Lice/nits may be found on visual inspection in this area.
  - Treatments of choice are topical pediculicides.
- Pediculosis corporis:
  - Presentation: widespread pruritus, usually involving the trunk.
  - Lice or nits may be found on clothing.
  - Treatment is to heat wash all clothing/linens in contact with infested person.
- Both scabies and pediculosis are primarily diagnosed clinically, based on characteristic physical findings and history. Biopsies or further testing are typically not necessary.

INTRODUCTION

Epidermal parasitic skin diseases are a category of infectious disease in which parasites are confined to the upper layer of the epidermis. The most commonly (worldwide) encountered epidermal skin diseases are scabies and pediculosis. Pediculosis may

Disclosure: The authors have nothing to disclose.
[a] Penn State Hershey Family Medicine Residency Program, Hershey, PA, USA; [b] Department of Family and Community Medicine, Penn State Milton S. Hershey Medical Center, Hershey, PA, USA; [c] Department of Orthopedics and Rehabilitation, Penn State Milton S. Hershey Medical Center, Hershey, PA, USA
[1] Present address: 121 Nyes Road, Suite A, Harrisburg, PA 17112, USA.
* Corresponding author. 121 Nyes Road, Suite F, Harrisburg, PA 17112.
E-mail address: jbutts@hmc.psu.edu

Prim Care Clin Office Pract 42 (2015) 661–675
http://dx.doi.org/10.1016/j.pop.2015.07.004
0095-4543/15/$ – see front matter © 2015 Elsevier Inc. All rights reserved.

be further subdivided into pediculosis capitis (head lice), pediculosis pubis (so-called crabs or pubic lice), and pediculosis corporis. There is a higher prevalence of many (but not all) of these infestations in lower socioeconomic populations and underprivileged conditions. Scabies and pediculosis corporis in particular are associated with lower socioeconomic status and crowded living conditions. Scabies has been estimated to have an occurrence rate as high as 46% in the developing world.[1] Pediculosis capitis was estimated to affect 1 in 4 school children in North America in 1997.

SCABIES
General Information and Cause

Scabies is a parasitic skin infestation by the mite, *Sarcoptes scabiei*. It is one of the most common parasitic skin infections, affecting approximately 300 million people worldwide.[2] *S scabiei* is a whitish-brown, 8-legged, turtle-shaped mite that measures approximately 0.4 × 0.3 mm, and is not grossly visible to the human eye (**Fig. 1**).

The female of the species is responsible for clinical manifestations of infestation. After fertilization by a male, the female mite burrows into the stratum corneum of the epidermis of a host and lay eggs. The female mite burrows about 2 mm into the epidermis each day, until reaching 10 to 25 mm below the surface. It lays 1 to 3 eggs each day for up to 1 to 2 months, after which the mite dies in the burrow. The eggs hatch in 3 to 4 days, the larvae then travel to the surface of the burrow, where they copulate, and fertilized females then continue this cycle.

Pathophysiology

The pruritus and rash occur as the result of a delayed type IV hypersensitivity reaction to mite proteins in mite saliva, scybala (feces), eggs, and the mite itself. For this reason, signs and symptoms of infestation, such as pruritus and rash, typically develop 3 to 4 weeks after primary exposure, or 1 to 2 days after reexposure.[3]

Risk Factors

Scabies are associated with resource-poor communities and lower socioeconomic status. It is more prevalent in overcrowded areas, and among populations with poor hygiene and inadequate living conditions. The elderly, the homeless, and sexually active young adults are at increased risk of exposure. People with pets that are not routinely bathed/cleaned may also be at some increased risk, although

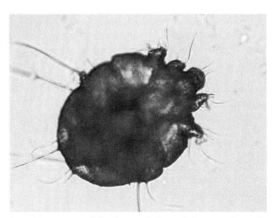

Fig. 1. *S scabiei* mite. (*Courtesy of* Professor Raimo Suhonen. DermNetNZ. Available at: http://www.dermnetnz.org.)

cross-species transmission of scabies is uncommon and even less likely to produce significant symptoms.

Transmission

Scabies is typically transmitted from direct person-to-person contact. Transmission to and from family members is common. Transmission at schools is uncommon because the level of contact that occurs in schools is not sufficient for the mites to travel to other hosts from an infected individual. In young adults, the most common method of transmission is sexual contact. Although uncommon, with higher parasite burdens, transmission can occur through fomite transmission. Contact with clothing or linens from an infected host, or on infected surfaces, such as a mattress or couch, is possible. Animals such as dogs and cats may also be vectors for scabies; however, the subspecies that infect these animals are distinct from the mites that infect humans. They are unable to reproduce on human hosts and rarely live longer than a few days. Infestations by them are therefore unlikely to cause extensive symptoms in humans.

Presentation

The most prominent symptom of scabies infection is pruritus and a skin rash. The pruritus begins about 3 to 4 weeks after infestation for primary exposures, and within 1 to 2 days for reexposures. The pruritus is often intense and typically worse at night. The skin rash appears as small, pruritic, erythematous papules. The distribution of these skin lesions in scabies is characteristic and typically involves the web spaces between the fingers, the flexor aspects of the wrists, the cubital fossa, the axillary folds, the periumbilical area, the waist, the area around the nipples, the extensor surfaces of the knees, the lateral and posterior aspects of the feet, and the genital area. The pathognomonic finding in scabies is the burrow made by the mites (**Fig. 2**).

It is typically seen as a thin reddish, brownish, or grayish line measuring from 2 to 15 mm long. However, burrows can be difficult to visualize because of their small size and also because they may be obscured by excoriations or crusting (from scratching).

Secondary staphylococcal or streptococcal infections are common and may complicate the clinical picture on presentation.

Because scabies is transmitted via direct skin-to-skin contact, clinicians should have a high index of suspicion if patients have come into contact with someone who may have scabies. Scabies occurs most often in the winter because mites survive longer on fomites and colder temperatures may predispose people to more crowded living conditions.

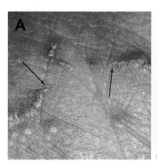 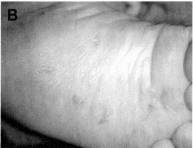

Fig. 2. Scabies burrows (*arrows*). ([*A*] *Courtesy of* Professor Raimo Suhonen. DermNetNZ. Available at: http://www.dermnetnz.org; and [*B*] *Courtesy of* DermNetNZ. Available at: http://www.dermnetnz.org.

Diagnosis

Scabies is typically a clinical diagnosis, based on the history and anatomic distribution of associated skin lesions. Finding burrows in the skin lesions on physical examination increases the certainty of diagnosis. Diagnostic tests such as skin scrapings, epidermal shave biopsy, adhesive tape test, and dermoscopy may also be used to provide more certainty in this diagnosis. However, negative results do not preclude the presence of scabies.[4] For this reason, a trial of scabicidal medication may be used both therapeutically and diagnostically; it is less invasive and time consuming than skin scraping or biopsy.

Skin scrapings and/or epidermal shave biopsies may be taken from high-yield areas and examined under low-power microscope for mites, mite droppings, and/or eggs.

Treatment

First-line treatment of scabies is topical permethrin 5% with 2 topical applications, 1 week apart. This cream should be massaged into the skin from the neck down to the soles of the feet, including the web spaces between fingers and toes. If lesions are present on the face, scalp, or neck, or in older patients or infants, permethrin may also be applied to the scalp and face.[5]

Oral ivermectin is also a reasonable first-line option. Recommended dosage is 200 µg/kg given twice, 2 weeks apart.

Second-line choices include topical crotamiton 10% cream and lindane 1% lotion. Although lindane is US Food and Drug Administration (FDA) approved for treatment of scabies in the United States, it has significant side effects, such as neurotoxicity, and therefore has been banned in several other countries. The FDA recommends caution with the use of lindane.

Topical steroids or systemic antihistamines may be given to reduce pruritus.

Clothing, linens, and bedding should be washed in hot water and dried at the hottest temperature setting in machine dryers to decontaminate them.

Complications

Secondary bacterial infection is common. Scabies is often considered a gateway infestation for new infections, especially *Staphylococcus* and *Streptococcus* species. There are several ways in which the scabies mite accomplishes this. The most overt is by making the skin barrier more vulnerable through direct breaks as it burrows through the skin.[6] However, recent studies have found that the mite, by secreting gut proteins, alters the microbiome of the skin to depress a host's immune response. This action not only allows the mite to better survive on hosts but also makes areas of infestation more prone to secondary infections.[7]

Prevention

To prevent transmission of scabies, it is recommended to examine and treat close contacts of infested persons, and to decontaminate clothing as noted earlier. Health care workers should also wear personal protective equipment such as gowns and gloves when dealing with infested patients. Maintaining good personal hygiene and regular bathing may also prevent or reduce transmission.

PEDICULOSIS
General Information

Pediculosis is an infestation of lice. Lice are obligate, ectoparasitic insects that feed on the blood of hosts. There are 3 main types of lice that are parasitic to humans, and each is responsible for a different variant of pediculosis infestation. Lice may infest the head (*Pediculus humanus capitis*), body (*Pediculus humanus corporis*), or pubic region (*Phthirus pubis*).[8]

PEDICULOSIS CAPITIS
Cause and Risk Factors

Of the 3 types of pediculosis infestation that affect humans, pediculosis capitis is the most common. There are an estimated 6 million to 11 million cases annually in the United States alone. Pediculosis capitis is caused by an infestation of the head and hair by the insect *P humanus capitis*, also called the head louse. This insect is a grayish white, blood-sucking parasite approximately 2 to 4 mm in length, with a flattened body and 3 pairs of legs that end in powerful claws that are used to grasp host skin and hair (**Fig. 3**).

The lifespan of a female louse is about 1 month, during which time a female can lay 7 to 10 eggs per day. Eggs are also known as nits. The eggs are firmly planted to the base of host hair shafts. They incubate and hatch in 7 to 12 days. Female lice grow for 9 to 12 days, then mate and lay more eggs. The life cycle of lice repeats every 3 to 4 weeks.

Pruritus occurs from a type IV hypersensitivity reaction to proteins in lice saliva, which are injected during feeding. Adult lice feed by sucking blood from the scalp and adjacent areas of the face and neck.

Risk factors for infestation include overcrowded living conditions, close contact (especially head-to-head contact) with infected people, and poor hygiene in adults who contract lice. Socioeconomic status, length of hair, and frequency of brushing and/or shampooing have not been shown to be risk factors for contracting this species of lice.[9]

Epidemiology

The Centers for Disease Control and Prevention (CDC) reports 6 to 12 million cases of pediculosis capitis in the United States annually. Lice infestations typically affect children aged 3 to 12 years more often than adults, regardless of hygiene. Girls also seem to be infested more often than boys. Infestations occur in all socioeconomic backgrounds. In the United States, African Americans are less frequently infected than white people, which is thought to be caused by geographic differences in lice claws,

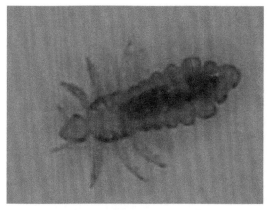

Fig. 3. *P humanus capitis.* (*Courtesy of* DermNetNZ. Available at: http://www.dermnetnz.org. Accessed November 28, 2014.)

with lice in North America being more adapted to grasping cylindrical hair (typically found on white people) as opposed to noncylindrical hair (more often seen in African Americans).

Transmission

Lice are wingless and unable to jump or leap from host to host. They can only survive for approximately 55 hours without a human host. In order for transmission to occur, they must crawl from one host to another during direct or close contact. In general, direct contact with the head or hair of an infected individual is required for transmission. Fomites such as clothing (hats, caps, scarves, and jackets), hair accessories (combs, brushes, ribbons, and barrettes), bedding, pillows, and towels have traditionally been implicated in transmission of pediculosis capitis; however, no clear evidence supporting this assertion exists.

Presentation

Lice infestation presents mainly with scalp, neck, and outer ear pruritus. However, infestation may also be asymptomatic, even in the setting of large infestations. Cervical and/or nuchal lymphadenopathy may be present. As with scabies, secondary bacterial infections are common. Adult lice or nits (eggs) attached to the proximal hair shafts may also be found on visual inspection. Nits appear as small white to yellow nodules firmly adhered to hair shafts (**Fig. 4**).

If a patient displays any of these characteristic symptoms it is important to ask about potential contacts with lice. For example, in the case of a child, it is appropriate to ask whether any cases of lice infestation were reported at the child's school, daycare, or summer camp.[10]

Diagnosis

The diagnosis is again a clinical diagnosis and may be made on physical examination by finding adult lice or viable nits attached to proximal hair shafts. Nits are often more easily visualized than adult lice. A Wood lamp may also be used to aid in diagnosis because nits fluoresce a pale blue color under this light. Nits may also be more easily visualized at the nape of the neck and behind the ears, just adjacent to the scalp.

Note that the presence of nits does not necessarily indicate an active lice infestation because nits can persist for months after successful treatment. The presence of many

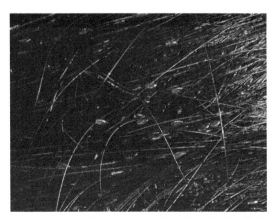

Fig. 4. Pediculosis capitis nits. (*Courtesy of* DermNetNZ. Available at: http://www. dermnetz.org. Accessed November 28, 2014.)

eggs within 6.5 mm (0.25 inch) of the scalp is suggestive of active infestation. Eggs found farther than 1 cm from the scalp are unlikely to be viable.

Treatment

The initial treatments of choice are topical pediculicides, such as pyrethroids (pyrethrin, permethrin), malathion, lindane, spinosad, dimethicone, or benzyl alcohol. When using topical pediculicides, patients should be cautioned not to use hair-conditioning products before use, because these may reduce the efficacy of topical pediculicides. Resistance to common pediculicides is emerging, so clinicians may need to find information on local resistance patterns to determine the optimal treatment. An important point for clinicians to keep in mind is that topical pediculicides target live lice but do not reliably kill their eggs. Repeat treatment based on the life cycle of lice (typically 7–10 days for eggs to hatch) is therefore recommended for full eradication.[11] Treatment options for pediculosis capitis are outlined in **Table 1**.

Nonpharmacologic treatment of pediculosis capitis involves moistening the hair with water, leaving conditioner in, and systematically combing the hair from root to tip with a lice comb. This method of wet combing may be preferred by some people who wish to avoid treatment with chemicals or medications. However, this involves considerable time because wet combing should be done every 3 days for 2 weeks. Even then, cure rates vary from 47% to 75%. Shaving the head has been anecdotally reported as an effective treatment of pediculosis capitis; however, no studies have been reported to evaluate this treatment method.

Complications

Rarely, scratching may lead to secondary bacterial infections on the scalp or face, such as impetigo. A reactive folliculitis may also occur as a result of either infestation or scratching, although it is also rare.

Prevention

It is recommended to avoid head-to-head contact with infested individuals. All household contacts of an infested person should be screened for lice and nits, and treated if infested. Even though the role of fomites in transmission of lice is unclear, current recommendations still favor avoidance of fomites. Sharing of clothing and hair accessories should be avoided. Lying or sitting in/on bedding/linens or furniture that was in contact with infested individuals until they are washed or cleaned should be avoided. Floors and furniture in the home of an infected individual should be vacuumed. Towels, linens, clothing, and bedding used or worn by infested individuals should be machine washed in hot water and dried in a high-temperature cycle before treatment, preferably in temperatures at or exceeding 54.4°C. Combs, brushes, and other plastic items may be soaked in hot water for 5 to 10 minutes to disinfect.

Some school districts have no-nit policies, under which children with nits are not permitted to attend school. The CDC recommends against this. School-aged children should not be restricted from school attendance because there is low risk of contagion in classrooms. Furthermore, the presence of nits does not indicate active infestation because nits can persist for months after successful treatment.

PEDICULOSIS PUBIS
Cause

Also known as crabs, this parasitic skin infection is caused by the crab louse, *P pubis* (**Fig. 5**).

Table 1
Treatment options for pediculosis capitis

Treatment	Mechanism and Use	Formulations/Brand Name	Application and Notes
Pyrethrins	• Neurotoxic • Pediculicidal • Reduced ovicidal effects on nits • Often combined with piperonyl butoxide for improved pyrethrin efficacy	Typically available as OTC lice shampoos with the following brand names: • Nix • Rid • Pronto • Clearlice	Use: • Wash hair with shampoo, rinse, and towel dry • Apply to damp hair and leave in for at least 10 min • Rinse off with water • A second application is indicated in 7–10 d to cover eggs hatched after initial application
Malathion	• Organophosphate cholinesterase inhibitor • Both pediculicidal and ovicidal	Malathion 0.5% lotion is available in the United States with a prescription and in the United Kingdom OTC An example brand name is Ovide	Use: • Apply to dry hair • Leave in place for 8–12 h • Wash with shampoo • Repeat application only if live lice are found 7–10 d after initial treatment Notes: • It is malodorous, sometimes to the point of irritation • A high alcohol content makes it flammable
Benzyl alcohol 5%	• A nonovicidal pediculicide • Mechanism is to obstruct the respiratory spiracles of live lice, leading to death by asphyxiation • May be used in patients aged 6 mo or older	Common brand name, available by prescription: • Ulesfia	Use: • Saturate dry scalp with the lotion • Leave in place for at least 10 min • Rinse off with water • This treatment should be repeated in 7–10 d Note: • Irritation of the skin, scalp, and eyes, and transient scalp numbness have been reported with this product
Spinosad 0.9%	• Neurotoxic pediculicide • FDA approved for pediculosis treatment in patients 4 y of age and older • Studies suggest it may be more efficacious than permethrin 1%	Common brand name, available by prescription: • Natroba	• Apply to dry hair • Completely coat the scalp and hair • Leave in place for at least 10 min • Rinse off with warm water

Lindane	• Neurotoxic pediculicide • No longer recommended as first-line therapy because of rare neurotoxic side effects in patients • Still FDA approved, with caution • Banned in the state of California as well as several countries • It should only be used as second-line treatment in refractory cases • Do not use in children, elderly, or adults weighing <50 kg (110 pounds) • Avoid in patients with skin conditions such as psoriasis or eczema because these may increase systemic absorption and thus neurotoxic side effects	Common brand name, available by prescription: • Kwell	Use: • Apply to scalp and hair • Leave in place for 4 min • Rinse with water Notes: • Apply with gloved hands to reduce systemic absorption • Gloves should be made of neoprene, nitrile, or vinyl; lindane is latex permeable • Dose should be no more than 57 g (2 ounces) • No more than 1 application is recommended
Ivermectin (topical)	• Neurotoxic pediculicide • It has both ovicidal and pediculicidal properties • A single application is typically sufficient	Common name brand, available by prescription: • Sklice	Use: • Coat the scalp and hair • Leave in place for at least 10 min • Rinse off with water Notes: • Topical ivermectin has been known to cause side effects of scalp and eye dryness and irritation
Ivermectin (oral)	• Neurotoxic pediculicide • Giving oral trimethoprim-sulfamethoxazole in conjunction with oral ivermectin may increase efficacy	Common brand name, available by prescription: • Stromectol • Recommended dose is 200 µg/kg	• Oral ivermectin is reserved for more refractory pediculosis infestations • Contraindicated in pregnant women and children weighing <15 kg
Dimethicone 4% lotion	• Not an insecticide • Clear odorless (synthetic silicone) gel that is thought to work against lice by coating and either asphyxiating them or disrupting water metabolism	Common brand names, available OTC: • Aveeno • LiceMD	Use: • Apply to dry hair and scalp • Leave in place at least 2 min • Comb lotion out • Do not shampoo hair for a least 8 h Notes: • Commonly found in OTC emollients such as Aveeno, usually as a 1% formulation • Stronger concentrations, such as 4%, found in products such as LiceMD are marketed as pediculicides

Abbreviation: OTC, over the counter.

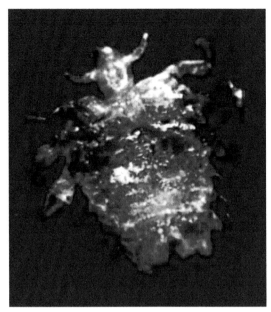

Fig. 5. *P pubis.* (*Courtesy of* DermNetNZ. Available at: http://www.dermnetnz.org. Accessed November 28, 2014.)

It is typically transmitted during sexual contact. Like many other parasitic skin infestations, the pruritus is a result of a type IV hypersensitivity reaction to louse saliva. The incubation period of phthiriasis is about 30 days, which corresponds with the 3-week to 4-week lifespan of the female louse. During that time, the female lays around 3 to 4 eggs (or nits) per day, potentially laying 26 eggs or more. Eggs are firmly attached to the bases of hairs (typically pubic hairs). The eggs hatch after 6 to 8 days and the cycle repeats.

Transmission

Direct contact is required for transmission. Like other lice species, *P pubis* is wingless and unable to jump or leap from host to host, and can only survive for about 55 hours without a human host. In order for transmission to occur, it must crawl from one host to another during direct, close contact. *P pubis* is typically transmitted during sexual contact. Although less common, transmission through fomites such as bedding/linen, clothing, and towels may also occur but, again, further studies are needed to fully evaluate the role of fomites in lice transmission.

Epidemiology

P pubis typically infests sexually active teenagers and young adults. The typical range is 15 to 40 years of age. Unlike in pediculosis capitis, *P pubis* seems to infest more men than women. Although infestation occurs in all socioeconomic classes, there is a greater prevalence of this louse in lower socioeconomic classes.

Presentation

Like other parasitic skin infestations, pubic lice also present with pruritus, most typically in the pubic area. However, *P pubis* can also attach to hairs in other areas, such as the axilla, abdomen, buttocks, perianal skin, and legs. In individuals with considerable body hair, no area of the body is immune to involvement, although the scalp is typically spared in most infestations. Some individuals develop small (<1 cm) macules on the skin. These macules are a sign of prolonged infestation and occur as a result of louse anticoagulant. Inguinal lymphadenopathy may also be present in infested individuals.

Although rare, crab lice can also attach to the eyelashes and eyebrows. This condition is known as phthiriasis palpebrarum. It is often misdiagnosed as blepharitis.[10] When seen in children, phthiriasis palpebrarum may be a sign of sexual abuse. Phthiriasis palpebrarum typically presents with intense pruritus of the eyelid and eyebrow margins. Infested individuals may complain of eye irritation as well. A reddish crusting and matting of the eyelashes may develop. It commonly presents with an associated conjunctivitis. Preauricular and submental lymphadenopathy may also be present. When present, signs/symptoms typically involve both eyes and eyelashes or eyebrows.

Diagnosis

Diagnosis is typically made from the physical examination and direct visualization of lice or nits. Nits may appear as small tannish nodules cemented to hair shafts (**Fig. 6**).

A magnifying lens or microscope may also be used to visualize lice/nits. As with pediculosis, a Wood lamp may also be used to aid in diagnosis because nits fluoresce a pale blue color under this light.[12]

Treatment

The CDC recommends treating phthiriasis with topical pediculicides plus combing out nits, then reevaluating patients in 9 to 10 days (**Table 2**).

Treatments for phthiriasis palpebrarum are modified to protect the eyes. First-line therapy is manual dislodging of the lice and nits and application of occlusive ophthalmic ointment to the affected area, twice a day for 10 days. Removal of the eyelashes may also be an option. One case series describes oral ivermectin as a reasonable second-line choice. Secondary conjunctivitis or infection may also need to be managed concurrently.[13]

In general, a second treatment may be required for full eradication 7 to 10 days after initial treatment, because most therapies are not reliably ovicidal. After 7 to 10 days, any viable nits should have hatched and the second treatment should eradicate the new lice.

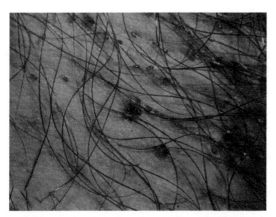

Fig. 6. *P pubis* nits. (*Courtesy of* DermNetNZ. Available at: http://www.dermnetnz.org. Accessed November 28, 2014.)

Table 2
Treatments for phthiriasis

Treatment	Mechanism and Use	Formulations/Brand Name	Application and Notes
First line: topical pyrethrins or permethrin (a synthetic pyrethrin)	• Neurotoxic and pediculicidal • Some ovicidal effects on nits	Common brand names, available OTC: • Nix • Rid • Pronto • Clearlice	• Cleanse and dry the hair • Apply to affected areas • Leave in place for 10 min • Wash in a manner similar to the treatment of pediculosis capitis
Second line: malathion 0.5%	• Organophosphate cholinesterase inhibitor • Pediculicidal and ovicidal	Available by prescription in the United States and OTC in the United Kingdom Common brand name: • Ovide	• Apply to affected area • Wash after 8–12 h
Oral ivermectin	• Neurotoxic pediculicidal, ovicidal	Common brand name, available by prescription: • Stromectol; 250 μg/kg in 2 doses, 2 wk apart	• Not for use in pregnant patients

Sexual contacts within a month of infestation should also be treated. Furthermore, clothing, bedding, towels, linen, and so forth should be decontaminated by machine washing in hot water and machine drying on the highest heat setting.

Patients should be advised to avoid sexual contact until the conclusion of their treatment, when there are no further signs of infection. Infested individuals should also be screened for other sexually transmitted diseases, because up to 30% of patients with pubic lice have been found to have 1 or more additional, concurrent sexually transmitted diseases.

Complications

Secondary bacterial infection is common. There is a higher prevalence of other concurrent sexually transmitted diseases in individuals infested with pediculosis pubis, so a thorough sexual history should be obtained.

Prevention

All recent sexual contacts should be treated in addition to the patient. Fomites should be decontaminated as noted previously.

PEDICULOSIS CORPORIS
Cause

P humanus corporis, or the body louse, is a 2-mm to 4-mm louse, slightly larger but similar in appearance and morphology to *P humanus capitis*. It typically inhabits a host's clothing, laying eggs along the seams. It crawls onto a host's skin to feed. As with all lice species that infest humans, symptomatic pruritus is caused by a type IV hypersensitivity reaction to louse saliva. It is not restricted to any particular area of the body, so patients may present with widespread symptoms. However, most pruritus typically involves the trunk. The body louse's life cycle is similar to that of head lice and pubic lice. Females live 3 to 4 weeks, during which time they lay eggs (nits) on the seams of hosts' clothing. Nits hatch after about a week, so total incubation time after initial infestation is about 1 month.[14]

Unlike the other 2 lice species that infest humans, *P humanus corporis* is a vector of transmission for other diseases (discussed later).

Epidemiology and Risk Factors

Pediculosis corporis is associated with resource-poor settings and poor personal hygiene. It is found mainly in colder climates and is virtually absent in the tropics. In industrialized nations, the body louse is most prevalent among the homeless population. Poverty, overcrowding, and poor personal hygiene are risk factors for this infestation. Other variables associated with infestation of the body louse are male gender, sleeping outdoors, and African American ethnicity.

Transmission

Like other lice species, *P humanus corporis* is wingless and unable to jump or leap from host to host, so direct close contact with infested individuals is required for transmission. However, unlike head or pubic lice, the body louse can survive for up to 3 days without a blood meal and does not infest host skin or hair, but clothing. Direct contact with fomites such as clothing is therefore a true vector for transmission of this louse.

Presentation

Like other lice infestations, pediculosis corporis presents with pruritus, although it may also be asymptomatic. The pruritus is typically widespread, but usually involves the trunk. Excoriations from scratching may also be present. Close inspection may reveal evidence of fresh bites, such as small hemorrhagic puncta or small papules. The areas of pruritus and excoriation may be most pronounced at the neck, axillary folds, and waist, where clothing most often comes into closest contact with skin.

Occasionally, lice or nits are found on body hair or skin; however, they are more likely to be visualized on inspection of clothing, in particular in and around the seams. To further complicate the clinical picture, secondary bacterial infection is common, as is concomitant bacterial infection from microbes for which the body louse is a vector. The body louse is a vector for diseases such as typhus, trench fever, relapsing fever, and plague. Many of these conditions are endemic to developing countries, and are not typically a major concern in industrialized nations.

Diagnosis

Diagnosis is clinical, typically made from the history and physical examination and direct visualization of lice or nits in/on a patient's clothing, especially the seams. Lice are occasionally found on the body, skin, or body hair, but inspecting the clothing is more likely to yield findings. Skin scrapings may be taken to differentiate from scabies, which presents with similar symptoms. Pediculosis corporis should be considered in the differentials for populations at higher risk of exposure, such as homeless individuals, or those with poor hygiene.[15]

Treatment

Because body lice typically inhabit clothing and not the skin/hair of hosts, the first-line treatment is different from other types of lice infestation. First-line treatment is to heat wash and heat dry all clothing and linens that were in contact with an infested individual, and for the infested individual to bathe thoroughly. Ironing or steam cleaning (dry cleaning) clothing with particular attention to the seams also kills lice. This treatment is sufficient for most infestations.

If a few lice or nits are found on the skin or body hairs, a topical pediculicide may also be used as outlined earlier in the treatment of pubic or head lice. Oral ivermectin has also been used because it has both pediculicidal and scabicidal activity, in case scabies is also suspected.

Low-potency topical steroids may be given after treatment of lingering symptoms of pruritus.

Complications

Pediculosis corporis is a vector for the bacteria *Rickettsia prowazekii* (typhus), *Borrelia recurrentis* (relapsing fever), *Bartonella quintana* (trench fever), and *Yersinia pestis* (plague). *B quintana* has been associated with endocarditis. Most of these diseases are typically associated with developing countries; however, coinfection with *B quintana* has been found in homeless populations in the United States and other industrialized countries. Many of these diseases present the possibility of serious infection and complications.[16,17]

Prevention

Good personal hygiene and washing clothing regularly are usually sufficient to prevent spread of this disease. Avoiding infested individuals and fomites is also recommended to prevent exposure.

SUMMARY/DISCUSSION

The most commonly encountered epidermal parasitic skin diseases are scabies and pediculosis. Both are primarily diagnosed clinically, based on characteristic physical findings and history. Fomites play a role in transmission. Important points to remember are that, in the case of scabies and pediculosis, children should not be excluded from school, because the level of contact that occurs there is typically not enough for transmission to occur. Current recommendations advise against no-nit policies at schools, for example. However, close contacts such as family members are at risk of transmission and screening these individuals for infestation is recommended. First-line treatment of scabies and pediculosis is topical antiparasitic agents. Systemic antiparasitic agents are available for more widespread or persistent infestations. Secondary infections from scratching are common in any epidermal parasitic skin infestation.

REFERENCES

1. Markova A, Kam SA, Miller DD, et al. Common cutaneous parasites. Ann Intern Med 2014;161(5). http://dx.doi.org/10.7326/0003-4819-161-5-201409020-01003.
2. Feldmeier H, Heukelbach J. Epidermal parasitic skin diseases: a neglected category of poverty-associated plagues. Bull World Health Organ 2009;87(2):152–9.
3. Rosamilia LL. Scabies. Semin Cutan Med Surg 2014;33(3):106–9.
4. Micali G, Lacarrubba F, Verzì AE, et al. Low-cost equipment for diagnosis and management of endemic scabies outbreaks in underserved populations. Clin Infect Dis 2015;60(2):327–9.
5. Centers for Disease Control and Prevention. Scabies, treatment. 2010. Available at: http://www.cdc.gov/parasites/scabies/treatment.html. Accessed November 28, 2014.

6. Morgan MS, Arlian LG, Markey MP. *Sarcoptes scabiei* mites modulate gene expression in human skin equivalents. PLoS One 2013;8(8):e71143.

7. Swe PM, Zakrzewski M, Kelly A, et al. Scabies mites alter the skin microbiome and promote growth of opportunistic pathogens in a porcine model. PLoS Negl Trop Dis 2014;8(5):e2897.

8. Do-Pham G, Monsel G, Chosidow O. Lice. Semin Cutan Med Surg 2014;33(3): 116–8.

9. Gunning K, Pippitt K, Kiraly B, et al. Pediculosis and scabies: a treatment update. Am Fam Physician 2012;86(6):535–41.

10. Feldmeier H. Treatment of pediculosis capitis: a critical appraisal of the current literature. Am J Clin Dermatol 2014;15(5):401–12.

11. Early J, MacNaughton H. Ivermectin lotion (Sklice) for head lice. Am Fam Physician 2014;89(12):984–6.

12. Yi JW, Li L, Luo da W. Phthiriasis palpebrarum misdiagnosed as allergic blepharoconjunctivitis in a 6-year-old girl. Niger J Clin Pract 2014;17(4):537–9.

13. El-Bahnasawy MM, Abdel FE, Morsy TA. Human pediculosis: a critical health problem and what about nursing policy? J Egypt Soc Parasitol 2012;42(3): 541–62.

14. Anane S, Malek I, Kamoun R, et al. Phthiriasis palpebrarum: diagnosis and treatment. J Fr Ophtalmol 2013;36(10):815–9.

15. Bonilla DL, Cole-Porse C, Kjemtrup A, et al. Risk factors for human lice and bartonellosis among the homeless, San Francisco, California, USA. Emerg Infect Dis 2014;20(10):1645–51.

16. Scanni G. Human phthiriasis. Can dermoscopy really help dermatologists? Entodermoscopy: a new dermatological discipline on the edge of entomology. G Ital Dermatol Venereol 2012;147(1):111–7.

17. Tomich EB, Knutson T, Welsh L. Hookworm-related cutaneous larva migrans. CJEM 2010;12(5):446.

Nail Deformities and Injuries

James Rory J. Tucker, MD

KEYWORDS

• Toenail • Deformities • Onychomycosis • Nail avulsion

KEY POINTS

- Nail deformities are common and easily detected by physical examination in an office setting by the primary care provider.
- Onychomycosis is highly prevalent and treatable in the primary care office setting. It causes prominent cosmetic disorder. Oral treatment duration can last 12 to 24 months and is capable of producing favorable results.
- To astute clinicians, a variety of systemic diseases, such as psoriasis, renal dysfunction, and iron deficiency, can present with nail findings.
- Nail avulsion is a simple procedure that can be performed in an outpatient office setting. For an ingrown toenail this procedure can provide immediate relief and eradication of the disorder.

NAIL ANATOMY

Nails offer protection for the dorsal aspects of fingers and toes and anatomically are composed of multiple parts. The most visible and recognizable nail segment is the nail plate, comprising what is commonly thought of as the nail. This structure is constructed largely of keratin, similar to hair, although of a different type. The plate is produced by the matrix, and multiple nail deformities result from altered keratinization at this location. Melanocytes are present in the matrix, but in a lower density than surrounding skin, giving nails their lighter color relative to the adjacent skin.[1] Surrounding the nail are the nail folds, with the cuticle at the proximal aspect. Deep to the nail plate is the nail bed. Proximally is the lunula, a lightly colored region so named for its shape. Fingernails grow about 1 cm in 3 months and toenails at about a third of this rate. Growth is slower on the nondominant hand and in old age.[2] See **Fig. 1** for a diagram of nail anatomy.

Disclosure: The author has nothing to disclose.
Department of Family and Community Medicine, Penn State Milton S. Hershey Medical Center, 500 University Avenue, Hershey, PA 17033, USA
E-mail address: jtucker@hmc.psu.edu

Prim Care Clin Office Pract 42 (2015) 677–691
http://dx.doi.org/10.1016/j.pop.2015.08.005
0095-4543/15/$ – see front matter © 2015 Elsevier Inc. All rights reserved.

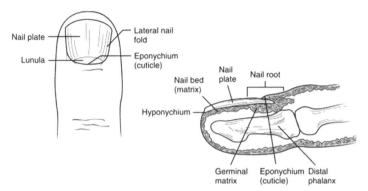

Fig. 1. Nail anatomy. (*From* Trott AT. The hand. In: Wounds and lacerations: emergency care and closure. 4th edition. Philadelphia: Saunders; 2012. p. 161–91; with permission.)

NAIL ABNORMALITIES
Onychomycosis

Fungal infection is the most common disease in ungual disorders, with a wide range of prevalence depending on geographic region.[1] Onychomycosis accounts for 40% to 50% of nail dystrophies. Risk factors for this infection include aging, diabetes, hemodialysis, poorly fitting shoes, and the presence of tinea pedis.[3,4] Transmission between family members is common and can be horizontal (eg, between spouses), or vertical between generations, which is more common than horizontal spread. Additional sources of infection are showers in locker rooms, public showers such as at pools, and mats in athletic facilities.[5] Intact skin serves as the primary barrier to infection. However, this may fail because of trauma or maceration.[3] Toenails are 25 times more likely than fingernails to be infected because of repeated blunt pressure from footwear.[6] Through this repetitive microtrauma, the distal edge of the nail is repeatedly lifted, giving opportunity for dermatophytes to establish residence.

Diagnosis of onychomycosis is made largely by physical examination. The primary part of the nail that is affected is the most distal, typically of the great toe. Assessment should be made regarding which part of the nail is involved, such as the nail plate distally, proximally, or the nail bed.[2] Distal onychomycosis is most common and can lead to thickening and yellowish discoloration (**Fig. 2**). Because the pharmacologic treatment of this can last up to 24 months, it is recommended to have definitive diagnosis before initiating treatment. Formal diagnosis can be made by testing nail scrapings using potassium hydroxide or pathology analysis of nail clippings.

Treatment can be difficult, with cure rates varying depending on the modality used. Topical treatment is available with ciclopirox nail lacquer 8% topical solution applied daily for 48 weeks, although, with eradication rates less than 50%, it is generally considered ineffective.[3,4] Oral treatment is recommended with either azoles or allylamines. The benefit of oral medications may not be visible for 12 months or longer because of infection being embedded within the nail plate and the slow growth rate of the nail. Common medications used include ketoconazole, itraconazole, terbinafine, and naftifine. Because of the prolonged duration of treatment required it is a good idea to know the patient's baseline liver function before beginning treatment.

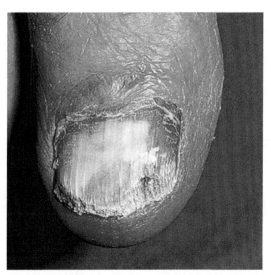

Fig. 2. Onychomycosis. (*From* White G, Cox N. Diseases of the skin. 2nd edition. St Louis (MO): Mosby; 2006; with permission.)

Leukonychia

Leukonychia is defined as discoloration of the nail with a white appearance (**Fig. 3**). Leukonychia can be classified as either true or apparent. True implies the discoloration originates within the matrix and emerges in the nail plate proper. If the disorder is exogenous to the nail plate, such as in superficial onychomycosis, it is termed pseudoleukonychia.[7] Apparent leukonychia looks as if the nail plate has whitened; however, this is caused by discoloration of the nail bed. This discoloration can occur if there is separation of the nail plate from the nail bed with an interspersed air space.[8] Discoloration of the nail plate can occur as a result of abnormal keratinization of the matrix and can be considered a normal variant for which no specific treatment is necessary.[4]

Some specific types of leukonychia are discussed here.

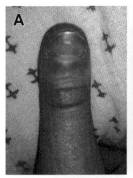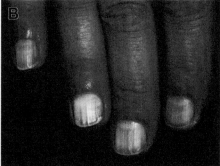

Fig. 3. (*A, B*) Examples of leukonychia. (*From* [A] Howard SR, Siegfried EC. A case of leukonychia. J Pediatr 2013;163(3):914–5; with permission; and [B] Pielasinski-Rodríguez Ú, Machan S, Fariña-Sabaris MC, et al. Acquired total leukonychia in a patient with human immunodeficiency virus infection. Actas Dermosifiliogr 2012;103(10):934–5, with permission.)

Mees lines

True leukonychia is caused by arsenic poisoning, and are characterized as transverse lines that may be single, multiple, and may involve multiple nails.[7] The lines migrate distally as the nail grows and indicate the time of arsenic intoxication by approximating 1 mm of growth from the cuticle per week (**Fig. 4**). Toenail concentrations of arsenic increase proportionally to exposure and can be measured at the tip approximately 100 days after initial exposure.[9]

Terry nails

Terry nails are apparent leukonychia with white nail proximally and normal color distally (**Fig. 5**).

Lindsay nail

Lindsay nail is the opposite of Terry nail, with a normal portion proximally and apparent leukonychia distally (**Fig. 6**). This condition may be seen in patients with chronic kidney disease or uremic renal failure.[7]

Muehrcke lines

Muehrcke lines are characterized by double white lines caused by apparent leukonychia (**Fig. 7**). These lines are caused by localized edema in the nail bed that exerts pressure on the vascular bed. These lines can be seen in renal disease, including nephrotic syndrome, glomerulonephritis, liver disease, and hypoalbuminemia.[4,7]

Melanonychia, Longitudinal

Hyperpigmented bands can occur as normal variants in black individuals. These bands must be differentiated from melanomas, for which personal and family history can be helpful, although ultimately a biopsy of the nail may be required (**Figs. 8** and **9**).[4]

Nail Pitting

Nail pitting typically results from defective keratinization in the matrix with parakeratotic cells in the superficial portion of the nail plate. These cells slough off from the nail plate and result in surface divots limited to the nail surface.[7,8] They may vary in

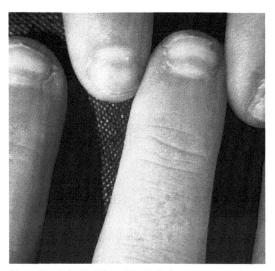

Fig. 4. Mees lines. (*From* Daniel CR, Scher RK. Nail changes secondary to systemic drugs or ingestants. J Am Acad Dermatol 1984;10(2 Pt 1):250–8; with permission.)

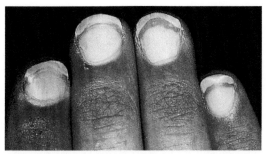

Fig. 5. Terry nails. (*From* Habif TP. Clinical dermatology: a color guide to diagnosis and therapy. 5th edition. St Louis: Mosby; 2010; with permission.)

size and have an irregular pattern, as in psoriasis, or a regular pattern, as in alopecia areata (**Fig. 10**).[2]

Subungual Hematoma

Subungual hematomas are produced as a result of trauma to the vascular structures within the nail bed. The mass of red or dark blood produces painful pressure as it accumulates (**Fig. 11**). Subungual hematomas can be easily drained using electrocautery to burn a small hole in the nail plate allowing the blood to drain. Alternatively, a large-

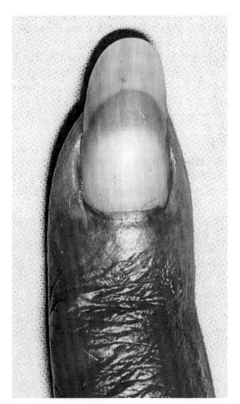

Fig. 6. Lindsay nails. (*From* Baliga RR. 250 cases in clinical medicine. 4th edition. Philadelphia, PA: Saunders, 2012; with permission.)

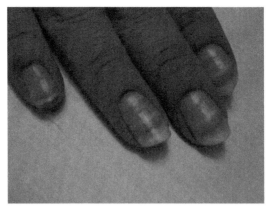

Fig. 7. Muehrcke lines. (*From* Short N, Shah C. Muehrcke's lines. Am J Med 2010;123(11):991–2; with permission.)

bore needle such as an 18-gauge can be used to drill a similar hole in the nail plate. If the hematoma involves greater than 50% of the nail plate, a nail bed laceration should be considered. If present, repair using primary intention may be necessary to ensure a favorable cosmetic result.[10]

Beau Lines

Transverse depressions in the nail are typically the result of severe illness and affect all 20 nails (**Fig. 12**). A single transverse depression limited to 1 digit can also occur because of localized trauma to the nail matrix as well as the nail. In either case, the depression is caused by temporary disruption of nail bed mitosis. This condition can be seen in individuals with Raynaud disease.[4] If the inciting event is significant enough to cause complete inhibition of nail formation for approximately 2 weeks, the depression will reach maximum depth, resulting in onychomadesis (**Fig. 13**).[7]

Onycholysis

Onycholysis is a common disorder involving distal nail plate separation from supporting structures such as nail bed, lateral nail fold, or hyponychium (**Fig. 14**). Discoloration of the nail can occur because of infection with *Pseudomonas* or *Candida*. Lifting of the

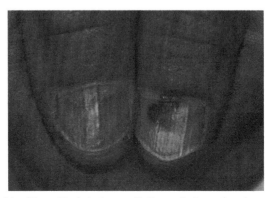

Fig. 8. Melanonychia. (*From* Finch J, Arenas R, Baran R. Fungal melanonychia. J Am Acad Dermatol 2012;66(5):830–41; with permission.)

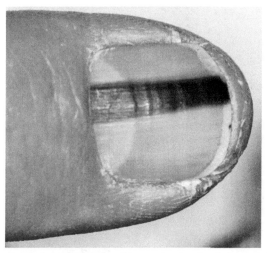

Fig. 9. Melanoma. (*From* Swartz MH. The skin. In: Textbook of physical diagnosis. 7th edition. Philadelphia: Elsevier Saunders; 2014. p. 81–144; with permission.)

distal nail plate can also be caused by trauma, particularly in individuals with long nails. The lifted nail plate is unlikely to reattach to the nail bed and the longer the duration of separation the lower the likelihood of reattachment because of keratinization of the exposed nail bed.[8] No specific treatment is required because the attached portion will continue to grow distally and the condition will be painless provided there is no further lifting of the nail.

Pterygium Unguis

In this condition the cuticle grows distally, distorting the proximal nail fold. It is typically caused by scarring loss of nail matrix. It may occur in the central portion, resulting in splitting of the nail, or progress to complete nail loss (**Fig. 15**).[2]

Longitudinal Ridging (Onychorrhexis)

Lines may appear as grooves or ridges and may represent systemic disease such as collagen vascular disease, protein deficiency, rheumatoid arthritis, or iron deficiency (**Fig. 16**).[7] If mild, this is commonly caused by brittle nails in advanced age.

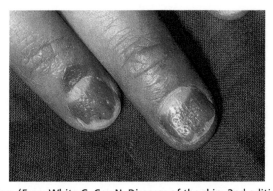

Fig. 10. Nail pitting. (*From* White G, Cox N. Diseases of the skin. 2nd edition. St Louis (MO): Mosby; 2006; with permission.)

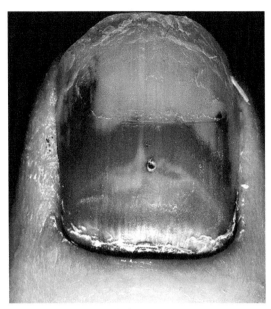

Fig. 11. Subungual hematoma. (*From* Habif TP. Nail diseases. In: Clinical dermatology. 6th edition. Philadelphia: Elsevier; 2016. p. 960–85; with permission.)

Trachyonychia

Commonly known as 20-nail dystrophy, this is a benign disease of the nail matrix. The inflammation caused by psoriasis and lichen planus can be traumatic to the nail matrix, causing a shift in keratinization. This shift is expressed as an altered nail plate, resulting in roughness of the nail plate like sandpaper (**Fig. 17**).[11]

Clubbing

Several features are characteristic in clubbing of the digits (**Figs. 18–20**). Notable are increased nail plate curvature in both the longitudinal and transverse planes, thickening of the nail bed soft tissue, positive Schamroth sign (absence of the space normally present at the proximal nail fold when nails are held in opposition), and Lovibond

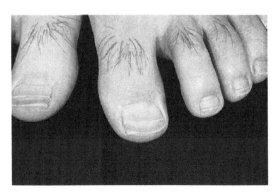

Fig. 12. Beau lines. (*From* Ferri FF. Diseases of the nails. In: Ferri's color atlas and text of clinical medicine. 1st edition. Philadelphia: Saunders; 2009. p. 76–83; with permission.)

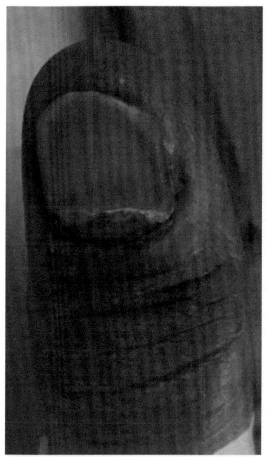

Fig. 13. Onychomadesis. (*From* Cashman MW, Sloan SB. Nutrition and nail disease. Clin Dermatol 2010;28(4):420–5; with permission.)

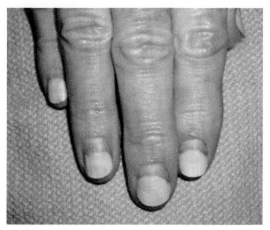

Fig. 14. Onycholysis. (*From* Vélez NF, Jellinek NJ. Simple onycholysis: a diagnosis of exclusion. J Am Acad Dermatol 2014;70(4):793–4; with permission.)

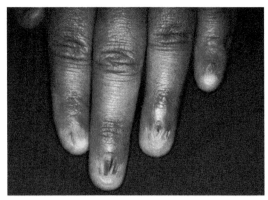

Fig. 15. Pterygium. (*From* Paller AS, Mancini AJ. Papulosquamous and Related Disorders. In: Hurwitz Clinical Pediatric Dermatology, 4th edition. Philadelphia, PA: Saunders, 2011. p. 71–91; with permission.)

angle greater than 180°. The Lovibond angle is measured at the junction of the nail plate and the proximal nail fold; it is normally less than 160°.[4,7,12] Greater than 80% of clubbing has cardiopulmonary causes, although clinicians should always be diligent in considering neoplastic cause.

Paronychia

Paronychia can occur as both an acute infection and as a chronic presentation. In the acute setting, it is an inflammatory reaction caused by bacterial invasion of the proximal or lateral nail fold. This condition presents as soft tissue swelling, erythema, and tenderness, with or without abscess formation (**Fig. 21**). Causative agents include *Staphylococcus aureus* and *Streptococcus pyogenes*.[4] In the absence of abscess formation, treatment with oral antibiotics with gram-positive coverage is reasonable. If the infection has progressed to the formation of an abscess, then incision and

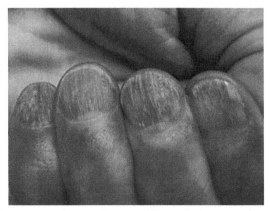

Fig. 16. Onychorrhexis. (*From* Thornton SL, Tomecki KJ. Nail Disease. In: Cleveland Clinic: current clinical medicine, 2nd edition. Philadelphia, PA: Saunders, 2010. p. 294–300; with permission.)

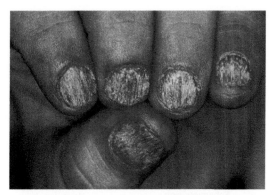

Fig. 17. Trachyonychia. (*From* Tosti A, Piraccini BM. Nail Disorders. In: Bolognia JL, Jorizzo JL, Schaffer JV, editors. Dermatology, 3rd edition. Elsevier: Saunders, 2012. p. 1129–47; with permission.)

drainage are required. In contrast, chronic paronychia typically lasts for longer than 6 weeks and is caused by *Candida* sp. This condition is generally seen in individuals with frequent extremity exposure to moisture, such as dishwashers.[4,13]

Ingrown Toenails

Ingrown nails commonly present to primary care clinicians. They can be a source of significant discomfort with ambulation for patients. Clinical presentation is similar to the presentation of paronychia, although location is limited to the lateral nail fold (**Fig. 22**). Causes of ingrown toenails are varied, but generally involve poorly fitting shoes, improper nail trimming, and genetic predisposition.[14] Toenails should be trimmed straight across with the edges extending distally of the lateral nail folds rather than curved into them (**Fig. 23**).

Conservative management should include a wide or open toe box to prevent pressure being applied to the lateral nail folds. In addition, soaking the affected toe or foot in warm soapy water before application of topical antibiotic provides relief.[15] If

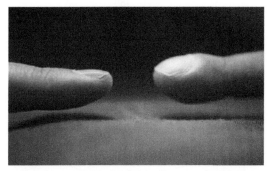

Fig. 18. Clubbing. (*From* Martínez-Lavín M, Pineda C. Digital clubbing and hypertrophic osteoarthropathy. In: Hochberg MC, Silman AJ, Smolen JS, et al, editors. Rheumatology, 6th edition. Philadelphia: Mosby, 2015; with permission.)

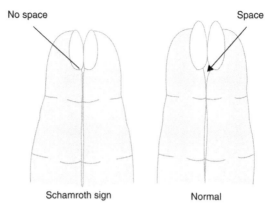

Fig. 19. Schamroth. (*From* Sainani G, Joshi VR, Sainani RG. Manual of clinical and practical medicine. 1st edition. New Delhi (India): Elsevier India; 2010; with permission.)

inflammation is significant or purulent drainage is evident, oral antibiotics with gram-positive coverage can be prescribed. Indications for a surgical avulsion, either full/complete or partial include, but are not limited to, the need to explore the nail bed or matrix, such as for laceration of the nail bed, glomus tumor, chronic parony-chia, chronic onychomycosis, or in the case of trauma to the nail warranting avulsion.

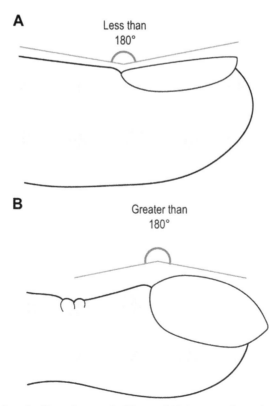

Fig. 20. Lovibond angle. (*From* Frowen P, O'Donnell M, Burrow JG, et al. Neale's disorders of the foot. 8th edition. London: Churchill Livingstone, Elsevier; 2010; with permission.)

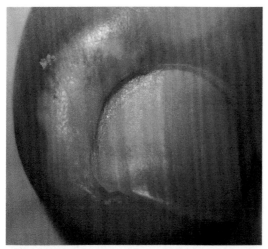

Fig. 21. Paronychia. (*From* Tosti A, Piraccini BM. Nail disorders. In: Bolognia JL, Jorizzo JL, Schaffer JV, editors. Dermatology. 3rd edition. Elsevier Saunders; 2012. p. 1129–47; with permission.)

Nail Avulsion Procedure

- A digital block is typically used for anesthesia, which can be in the form of a ring block or 2 vertical injections medial and lateral to the proximal phalange.
- Using 2% lidocaine rather than 1% allows less discomfort caused by volume distension.
- It is common practice to avoid the use of epinephrine because of fear of tissue necrosis. However, this is debatable.[16]
- Use of a toe tourniquet is at the discretion of the health care provider.
- With a periosteal elevator, Freer elevator, or blunt edge of surgical scissors, the nail plate is detached from the nail bed using firm pressure. If performing partial nail avulsion it is only necessary to detach the involved one-third of the nail then, using a pair of scissors, the nail is cut from its distal edge proximally, all the way to its origin at the germinal matrix.
- With a hemostat, the affected nail is twisted edge up and out of the lateral nail fold.
- After complete detachment from the nail bed, continuous traction is applied distally to remove the nail or nail segment from its proximal attachment.
- The germinal nail matrix is ablated using electrocautery or phenol.
  - Electrocautery requires a dry surface to function.
  - Phenol solution should be applied in 2 to 3 cycles of 30-second applications.
  - When complete, the phenol is neutralized with isopropyl alcohol to minimize tissue damage.
- A nonadherent, absorbent dressing is applied, because oozing is to be expected and is possible for up to 6 weeks.[15]
- The patient should be advised to remain in limited weight bearing status for the remainder of the day.
- Dressings may be removed after 24 hours and the toe should be soaked in warm water twice a day.
- The patient may return to wearing shoes on day 3.
- Gradual return to full activity over 1 week, as tolerated.

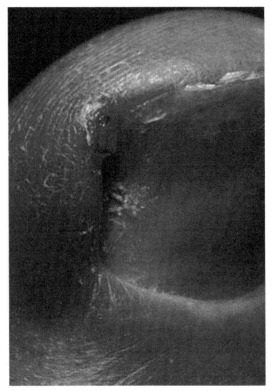

Fig. 22. Ingrown nail. (*From* Habif TP, Campbell JL, Chapman MS, et al. Hair and nail diseases. In: Skin disease: diagnosis and treatment. 3rd edition. Philadelphia: Saunders; 2011. p. 562–89; with permission.)

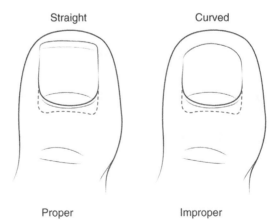

Fig. 23. Proper toenail trimming. (*From* McGee DL. Podiatric procedures. In: Roberts JR, editor. Roberts and Hedges' clinical procedures in emergency medicine. 6th edition. Philadelphia: Saunders; 2014. p. 1028–41; with permission.)

SUMMARY

A diversity of nail deformities is easily detectable by clinicians in an office setting. Several are benign and a basic knowledge of nail anatomy and these physical findings enables providers to determine when to reassure the patient and when a more detailed evaluation is required. In addition, clinicians should be comfortable offering nail avulsion in their offices when the circumstances call for this procedure.

REFERENCES

1. Fernandez-Flores A, Saeb-Lima M, Martínez-Nova A. Histopathology of the nail unit. Rom J Morphol Embryol 2014;55(2):235–56.
2. Wright A. ABC of dermatology. Br Med J 1988;296:106–9.
3. Hainer B. Dermatophyte infections. Am Fam Physician 2003;67(1):101–8.
4. Tully A, Trayes K. Evaluation of nail abnormalities. Am Fam Physician 2012;85(8): 779–87.
5. Nenoff P, Krüger C, Ginter-Hanselmayer G, et al. Mycology–an update. Part 1: Dermatomycoses: causative agents, epidemiology and pathogenesis. J Dtsch Dermatol Ges 2014;12:188–209.
6. Kaur R, Kashyap B, Bhalla P. Onychomycosis–epidemiology, diagnosis and management. Indian J Med Microbiol 2008;26(2):108–16.
7. Singal A, Arora R. Nail as a window of systemic diseases. Indian Dermatol Online J 2015;6(2):67–74.
8. Jadhav V, Mahajan P, Mhaske C. Nail pitting and onycholysis. Indian J Dermatol Venereol Leprol 2009;75(6):631–3.
9. Das N, Sengupta S. Arsenicosis: diagnosis and treatment. Indian J Dermatol Venereol Leprol 2008;74(6):571–81.
10. Wang Q, Johnson B. Fingertip injuries. Am Fam Physician 2001;63(10):1961–6.
11. Gordon K, Vega J, Tosti A. Trachyonychia: a comprehensive review. Indian J Dermatol Venereol Leprol 2011;77(6):640–5.
12. Singh G. Nails in systemic disease. Indian J Dermatol Venereol Leprol 2011; 77(6):646–51.
13. Grinzi P. Hair and nails. Aust Fam Physician 2011;40(7):476–84.
14. Ogur R, Tekbas O, Hasde M. Managing infected ingrown toenails: longitudinal band method. Can Fam Physician 2005;51:207–8.
15. Khunger N, Kandhari R. Ingrown toenails. Indian J Dermatol Venereol Leprol 2009;78(3):279–89.
16. Pandhi D, Verma P. Nail avulsion: indications and methods (surgical nail avulsion). Indian J Dermatol Venereol Leprol 2012;78(3):299–308.

United States Postal Service
Statement of Ownership, Management, and Circulation
(All Periodicals Publications Except Requestor Publications)

1. Publication Title
Primary Care: Clinics in Office Practice

2. Publication Number
0 4 4 - 6 9 9 0

3. Filing Date
9/18/15

4. Issue Frequency
Mar, Jun, Sep, Dec

5. Number of Issues Published Annually
4

6. Annual Subscription Price
$225.00

7. Complete Mailing Address of Known Office of Publication *(Not printer)(Street, city, county, state, and ZIP+4®)*
Elsevier Inc.
360 Park Avenue South
New York, NY 10010-1710

Contact Person
Stephen R. Bushing

Telephone *(Include area code)*
215-239-3688

8. Complete Mailing Address of Headquarters or General Business Office of Publisher *(Not printer)*
Elsevier Inc., 360 Park Avenue South, New York, NY 10010-1710

9. Full Names and Complete Mailing Addresses of Publisher, Editor, and Managing Editor *(Do not leave blank)*

Publisher *(Name and complete mailing address)*
Linda Belfus, Elsevier Inc., 1600 John F. Kennedy Blvd., Suite 1800, Philadelphia, PA 19103

Editor *(Name and complete mailing address)*
Jessica McCool, Elsevier Inc., 1600 John F. Kennedy Blvd., Suite 1800, Philadelphia, PA 19103-2899

Managing Editor *(Name and complete mailing address)*
Adrianne Brigido, Elsevier Inc., 1600 John F. Kennedy Blvd., Suite 1800, Philadelphia, PA 19103-2899

10. Owner *(Do not leave blank. If the publication is owned by a corporation, give the name and address of the corporation immediately followed by the names and addresses of all stockholders owning or holding 1 percent or more of the total amount of stock. If not owned by a corporation, give the names and addresses of the individual owners. If owned by a partnership or other unincorporated firm, give its name and address as well as those of each individual owner. If the publication is published by a nonprofit organization, give its name and address.)*

Full Name	Complete Mailing Address
Wholly owned subsidiary of	1600 John F. Kennedy Blvd, Ste. 1800
Reed/Elsevier, US holdings	Philadelphia, PA 19103-2899

11. Known Bondholders, Mortgagees, and Other Security Holders Owning or Holding 1 Percent or More of Total Amount of Bonds, Mortgages, or Other Securities. If none, check box ☑ None

Full Name	Complete Mailing Address
N/A	

12. Tax Status *(For completion by nonprofit organizations authorized to mail at nonprofit rates) (Check one)*
The purpose, function, and nonprofit status of this organization and the exempt status for federal income tax purposes:
☐ Has Not Changed During Preceding 12 Months
☐ Has Changed During Preceding 12 Months *(Publisher must submit explanation of change with this statement)*

13. Publication Title
Primary Care: Clinics in Office Practice

14. Issue Date for Circulation Data Below
September 2015

PS Form 3526, July 2014 [Page 1 of 3 (Instructions Page 3)] PSN 7530-01-000-9931 PRIVACY NOTICE: See our Privacy policy in www.usps.com

---

15. Extent and Nature of Circulation *(Net press run)*

			Average No. Copies Each Issue During Preceding 12 Months	No. Copies of Single Issue Published Nearest to Filing Date
a.	**Total Number of Copies** *(Net press run)*		206	183
b. Legitimate Paid and Or Requested Distribution (By Mail and Outside the Mail)	(1)	Mailed Outside County Paid/Requested Mail Subscriptions stated on PS Form 3541. *(Include paid distribution above nominal rate, advertiser's proof copies and exchange copies)*	100	90
	(2)	Mailed In-County Paid/Requested Mail Subscriptions stated on PS Form 3541. *(Include paid distribution above nominal rate, advertiser's proof copies and exchange copies)*		
	(3)	Paid Distribution Outside the Mails Including Sales Through Dealers And Carriers, Street Vendors, Counter Sales, and Other Paid Distribution Outside USPS®	24	27
	(4)	Paid Distribution by Other Classes of Mail Through the USPS (e.g. First-Class Mail®)		
c.	**Total Paid and or Requested Circulation** *(Sum of 15b (1), (2), (3), and (4))*	▲	124	117
d. Free or Nominal Rate Distribution (By Mail and Outside the Mail)	(1)	Free or Nominal Rate Outside-County Copies included on PS Form 3541	16	10
	(2)	Free or Nominal Rate In-County Copies included on PS Form 3541		
	(3)	Free or Nominal Rate Copies mailed at Other classes Through the USPS (e.g. First-Class Mail®)		
	(4)	Free or Nominal Rate Distribution Outside the Mail *(Carriers or Other means)*	16	10
e.	**Total Nonrequested Distribution** *(Sum of 15d (1), (2), (3) and (4))*	▲	16	10
f.	**Total Distribution** *(Sum of 15c and 15e)*	▲	140	127
g.	**Copies not Distributed** *(See instructions to publishers #4 (page #3))*		66	56
h.	**Total** *(Sum of 15f and g)*	▲	206	183
i.	**Percent Paid and/or Requested Circulation** *(15c divided by 15f times 100)*		88.57%	92.13%

* If you are claiming electronic copies go to line 16 on page 3. If you are not claiming Electronic copies, skip to line 17 on page 3.

16. Electronic Copy Circulation		Average No. Copies Each Issue During Preceding 12 Months	No. Copies of Single Issue Published Nearest to Filing Date
a. Paid Electronic Copies	▲		
b. Total Paid Print Copies *(Line 15c)* + Paid Electronic copies *(Line 16a)*	▲		
c. Total Print Distribution *(Line 15f)* + Paid Electronic Copies *(Line 16a)*	▲		
d. Percent Paid *(Both Print & Electronic copies)* *(16b divided by 16c X 100)*	▲		

☐ I certify that 50% of all my distributed copies (electronic and print) are paid above a nominal price

17. Publication of Statement of Ownership
If the publication is a general publication, publication of this statement is required. Will be printed in the __December 2015__ issue of this publication.

18. Signature and Title of Editor, Publisher, Business Manager, or Owner

Stephen R. Bushing

Stephen R. Bushing – Inventory Distribution Coordinator

Date
September 18, 2015

I certify that all information furnished on this form is true and complete. I understand that anyone who furnishes false or misleading information on this form or who omits material or information requested on the form may be subject to criminal sanctions (including fines and imprisonment) and/or civil sanctions (including civil penalties).

PS Form 3526, July 2014 (Page 3 of 3)

Moving?

Make sure your subscription moves with you!

To notify us of your new address, find your **Clinics Account Number** (located on your mailing label above your name), and contact customer service at:

Email: journalscustomerservice-usa@elsevier.com

800-654-2452 (subscribers in the U.S. & Canada)
314-447-8871 (subscribers outside of the U.S. & Canada)

Fax number: 314-447-8029

Elsevier Health Sciences Division
Subscription Customer Service
3251 Riverport Lane
Maryland Heights, MO 63043

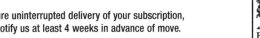
ELSEVIER

Printed and bound by CPI Group (UK) Ltd, Croydon, CR0 4YY

03/10/2024

01040494-0007